THE
7-DAY
BELLY
MELT
DIET

G

GALVAN!ZED
Media

This book proposes a program of diet and exercise recommendations for the reader to follow. However, you should consult a qualified medical professional (and, if you are pregnant, your ob-gyn) before starting this or any other diet or fitness program. Please seek your doctor's advice before making any decisions that affect your health or extreme changes in your diet, particularly if you suffer from any medical condition or have any symptom that may require treatment. As with any diet or exercise program, if at any time you experience discomfort, stop immediately and consult your physician.

Mention of specific companies, organizations, or authorities in this book does not imply endorsement by the author or publisher, nor does mention of specific companies, organizations, or authorities imply that they endorse this book, its author, or the publisher.

Copyright © 2018 by Galvanized Media, LLC

All rights reserved.

Distributed by Simon & Schuster

ISBN 978-1-940358-25-3
Ebook ISBN 978-1-940358-28-4

Printed in the United States of America on acid-free paper.

Design by Andy Turnbull

THE
7-DAY
BELLY
MELT
DIET

The scientifically proven plan to flatten your stomach and keep you lean for life.

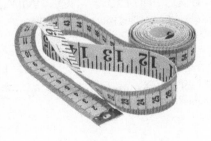

By the Editors of
Eat This, Not That!®

Contents

THE 7-DAY BELLY MELT DIET

INTRODUCTION

Strip Away Fat Superfast

ALL YOUR LIFE you've been told that good things come to those who wait. Be patient. As long as you stay within the lines, obey the rules, take your time, and work hard—for months, years, decades—you'll eventually see results.

When it comes to weight loss, you've probably heard the same spiel: Take it slow, set realistic goals, don't get ahead of yourself. There are speed limits in life, and you need to obey them.

But what if there's no time to wait? And what if taking the path of the tortoise isn't the most effective or efficient route to your destination?

For losing weight and shedding belly fat, new research suggests that patience isn't a virtue. It may actually be a mistake—especially if your high school reunion is just three weeks away!

Those OMG Moments!

Let's see if you can relate to these three stressful dieting deadlines:

21 DAYS: It's just three weeks until your high school reunion, and you've got to resemble your Facebook photo, you know, the one that's four years old!

14 DAYS: You want to look good for that family wedding in two weeks and you wish there was some way you could shed 20 pounds without dropping everything and joining an emergency fat-loss boot camp.

7 DAYS: You have a job interview with a great company and you know that first impressions count. Or your beach vacation is just a week away and your reflection in the mirror leaves no doubt that the sexy swimsuit you were hoping to wear will not fit. Not even close.

Do any of those fire drills sound familiar?

How many times have you looked at the calendar and felt a knot tighten in your belly when you notice a rapidly advancing social event and realize—*OMG, I'm going to be with people who matter to me who haven't seen me in a year!*

We know. You shouldn't worry about how people perceive you based on how you look on the outside. It's who you are inside that matters. Of course! But we all care about how we appear to others. There's nothing wrong with that. It's natural to want to look fit and healthy and attractive, especially on important occasions or during those times when shorts, swimsuits, and spaghetti straps will reveal body parts that might normally be hidden from view. There's no shame in wanting to shape up and see visual results quickly because, well, the high school reunion *is* right around the corner. And *you know who* will be there...

Fortunately, for those who follow The 7-Day Belly Melt Diet, it's the hare, not the tortoise, that wins the race. Today's science tells us that all those slow and steady, easy as she goes diet plans simply aren't practical for most people. The best way to lose pounds, especially from the abdominal region, and improve your health NOW isn't to go slow. It's to break the rules, ignore the speed limit, and race through every traffic light that gets in your way. Fast, astounding results can be yours.

The 7-Day Belly Melt Diet is going to show you how to strip away pounds with lightning speed, and prove why moving quickly is your very best chance for staying slim and healthy for years to come. In fact, this approach is so unconventional—and flies so dramatically in the face of everyday "slow and steady" wisdom—that the people in your life are going to be astounded by how quickly your body changes.

You'll be astounded, too.

Take the Fast Lane to Slim City

There's a reason that slow and steady weight loss has been the preferred approach of so many health professionals: The traditional belief has been that to lose weight and keep it off you need to make gradual lifestyle changes. By slowly getting used to a new way of eating and living, you won't shock your body too drastically, and over time, those changes will become permanent. Plus, we've all been warned about the dangers of yo-yo dieting; ever since the days when a slim-me-down Oprah dragged that little red wagon of fat around the studio then later wound up putting it right back onto her body, we've been aware that losing weight in dramatic fashion often means gaining it all back, and then some.

Except, sometimes common sense turns out to be common nonsense. And when it comes to weight loss, the science now tells us that dropping pounds shouldn't be a marathon, but rather a 100-yard dash.

Not long ago, when researchers conducted a comprehensive review of weight-loss studies, they discovered that people who lost weight the fastest were the most likely to keep it off in the long run. "Regardless of whether you pick a sensible diet, exercise, behavioral therapy, or a drug, our analysis of the literature shows that it's those who experience the greatest weight loss in the first two to four weeks who have the greatest weight loss the following year," wrote Arne Astrup, a researcher at Copenhagen University's Department of Nutrition, Exercise and Sports, who helped put together the analysis. "So if you've lost a lot of weight after one month, you're more likely to have lost a lot of weight after a year or two."

In one example, Astrup and his team reviewed a study of two sets of obese people who underwent very different diet programs: One led to rapid weight loss, while the other produced slow and steady results. For the purposes of their review, published in the *New England Journal of Medicine,* "rapid weight loss" meant dropping around one kilo—or a little over two pounds—per day. It turned out that those who lost weight slowly fared no better in the long run than those who lost weight quickly. In fact, the slow loss group was more likely to lose motivation sooner.

Think about that: Your best chance of losing your belly and keeping it off for good is to lose more than two pounds a day! That means your goal should be to strip off eight pounds in the next four days! Or 14 pounds in seven days. Even if your weight loss happens to slow down a bit after the initial weeks of following a new eating and lifestyle program (this is typical as you become leaner and fitter), you could expect to drop 30, 35, 40 pounds or even more in a month! Don't think you can lose that much that quickly? Even if you expected a more conservative weight loss of, say, 10 pounds in 7 days—a little more than a pound a day—wouldn't you be happy with that?

We think so. That kind of weight loss will not only shock you and the people around you, but it will set you up for a lifetime of better health, greater happiness, and a leaner, lighter, stronger physique.

And it's totally realistic. Very doable. Your first step is to discard the old thinking about how to lose weight and to embrace the power of speed.

OLD THINKING:
Set realistic goals.

NEW PLAN:
Be ambitious!

Several studies have shown that more ambitious goals are often associated with better weight-loss outcomes. In fact, Astrup found that when weight-loss experts intervene and encourage dieters to set more realistic weight-loss goals they don't actually shed the weight they want and keep it off any longer than dieters who target bigger and faster weight loss. In other words, there are downsides to being conservative, heavy ones.

OLD THINKING:
Lose weight slowly, stay slim for life.

NEW PLAN:
Lose weight rapidly, stay slim for life.

You're more than five times as likely to succeed in your long-term weight-loss goals if you start dropping pounds rapidly right out of the gate, according to a 2013 study in the *International Journal of Behavioral Medicine*. The same results have been repeated over and over. A 2014 study in *The Lancet* looked at 200 people on diet plans and found that "achieving a weight loss target of 12.5 percent [of body weight] is more likely, and dropout is lower, if losing weight is done quickly." And a similar study in the *Journal of Nutrition Education and Behavior* found that subjects who were more successful in the initial weeks of a weight-loss program were far more likely to stay motivated, and go on to lose at least 5 percent of their body weight, than those who started more slowly.

OLD THINKING:

You need to prepare yourself for diet success.

NEW PLAN:

Don't wait; start right now!

You can't lose weight by planning to lose weight. That's called procrastination. Don't delay. Don't overthink this. Start today. Bookmark this page and then jump over to page 20 where you will find the 7-Day Belly Melt Diet Contract. Sign and date it. It's a promise to yourself that signals your commitment to following the diet program.

Why do we ask you to sign this symbolic contract? Well, it marks a definitive break between your old lifestyle and your adoption of a new mind-set for healthier eating and living. Besides, studies show that the act of making a promise to yourself improves your chances of sticking to it. You make it even harder to compromise your commitment by making your intentions public.

So sign that document and celebrate with a tall glass of ice water, not with some sugary soda or juice. That's another positive step you can take right now with immediate benefits. On this program, you will be eliminating the source of at least 25 percent of your daily calories—empty calories from sugary beverages.

Burn 3,500 calories, drop one pound.

Eat right, weigh less.

You've probably heard some version of what scientists refer to as the 3,500 kcal rule: A pound of fat is equal to 3,500 calories. Thus, says the rule, by eliminating 3,500 calories from your body through a combination of consuming fewer calories and burning off more through physical activity, you can expect to drop one pound. This idea, developed more than half a century ago, is as set in stone as the Ten Commandments, and even the American Medical Association abides by it. But more and more, we're learning that it's simply not true: Some people will lose a pound of body weight without creating that 3,500 calorie deficit. And some people won't be able to lose a pound no matter how hard they work to burn off those calories.

The fact is, our bodies adapt to new exercise regimens really quickly, and research from the Pennington Biomedical Research Center in Baton Rouge, Louisiana, indicates that when it comes to exercise, over the long run, our bodies actually lose weight at about one third the rate we once thought. So you could jog away an extra 500 calories a day and expect to lose a pound a week (7 days X 500 calories = 3,500 calories), but in reality, you'd probably lose much less than that.

That's actually good news. After all, who wants to jog every day for a week to lose a mere pound? We've got a better way!

OLD THINKING:

You need to sweat for 30 minutes or more during a workout to get anything from exercise.

NEW PLAN:

Do our quick, efficient workouts and get on with your life.

We've rounded up the scientific proof that very brief exercise sessions can be incredibly beneficial to your health, improving cardiovascular function and insulin resistance and triggering weight loss. In this book, you'll find exercise sessions that can fit into any schedule, no matter how busy you are. In Chapter 11, we give you 6-minute, 10-minute, 15-minute, and 30-minute exercise plans that you can do at home without special equipment. There's even a One Minute Morning Energizer to jump-start your metabolism each day that we suggest you do in the bathroom before you have your coffee.

OLD THINKING:

You need to be physically fit in order to start losing weight.

NEW PLAN:

It doesn't matter if you're "in shape." Just get moving!

Maybe you weren't very good at sports as a kid. So what? The exercises in this book aren't crazy-hard. Maybe you haven't exercised in years. That's okay, too. You can be in terrible shape and still lose that belly. Two meta-analyses found that even when schools offered students specialized gym classes designed to help them cope with obesity, the students' fitness at the beginning of the program made no difference in their longterm weight-loss success. Prepping yourself to "get fit" doesn't matter at all; what matters is that you're ready to start losing weight right now. The fitness will come naturally.

OLD THINKING:
Everything in moderation.

NEW PLAN:
Rapid weight loss means sticking to a serious meal plan that works.

A 2015 study at the Friedman School of Nutrition Science and Policy at Tufts University found that while most doctors subscribe to the notion of "all things in moderation," that longstanding general advice is actually wrong. When researchers looked at the diets of 6,814 people, they found that the more diverse a person's diet, the more likely he or she was to experience weight gain. In fact, the test subjects who ate the widest range of foods showed a 120 percent greater increase in waist circumference compared with those who had the least diversity. In other words, people who have the best success at weight loss don't follow the "everything in moderation" advice, but choose specific healthy foods to focus on and tend to stick to them.

Everything in moderation sounds good, but it can backfire on you because the "in moderation" part is so challenging to pull off. Think about it: Pull a pint of chocolate ice cream out of your freezer and grab a spoon. Have just one tablespoon. Okay, you can have two. That's still a moderate amount. Now stop. That's all you get. Put the ice cream pint back and step away from your fridge. Hard to

Get Off the Noodle Roller-Coaster
Eating pasta makes you hungry for more pasta.

Have you ever had spaghetti with tomato sauce and a hunk of garlic bread—and gone back for seconds? When you consume a lot of carbs, especially dough-based carbs made with white flour, your blood sugar increases, which triggers your pancreas to churn out a lot of insulin. That sugar-regulating hormone drives down your blood sugar, and you become ravenously hungry again.

People who eat a lot of bread and pasta tend to be overweight. A recent Spanish study of more than 9,000 people compared the body composition of those who ate two or more servings of white bread per day to that of those who ate less and found that the heavy carb eaters were 40 percent more likely to become overweight or obese. Even eating whole-wheat pasta (which contains more fiber than regular pasta) may make you hungrier. Not all whole grains are equally filling, either, according to a study in *The Journal of the Federation of American Societies for Experimental Biology*. In an experiment, researchers found that people who ate wheat became hungry significantly sooner afterward compared with people who ate an equal portion of barley.

do, no? And it's easy to justify opening up the freezer again because what harm can come from another bite or two of ice cream? That's still in moderation, right?

This is an important point: By simplifying your diet—that is, reducing your food choices—you make it easier to eat healthfully and lose weight because you limit those foods (like ice cream) that are so difficult to eat in moderation.

Probably the most significant and challenging dietary change you'll make during this 7-day program is cutting out white bread, pasta, white rice, and other highly processed grains. You can eat some whole grains, but we would like you to limit those to whole-grain crackers, an occasional whole-grain bun or slice of sandwich bread, and a little bit of brown rice or quinoa with dinner once or twice during your 7-day plan. Why so little whole grains? Because pastas and breads are where most people unconsciously overindulge—even when they stick to the higher-in-fiber whole-grain kind.

The 7-Day Belly Melt Diet is designed to show you that you can eat incredibly delicious foods and feel satisfied without relying on bread, pasta, and rice. This is a learning process, and the goal is to demonstrate the power of cutting way back on these carbohydrates so that you don't have to banish them forever (what fun is that?) but can eat them mindfully, which means not often. By following our simple plan of limited food variety and adhering to a few sound nutrition rules, your belly will melt away—rapidly. And you'll recognize how building your meals around grains (think pasta and rice dishes, and bread-heavy recipes), as many people do, can put the weight on (or put lost pounds right back on).

Simplicity is a very powerful weight-loss tool. Limiting your food choices makes life simpler and weight loss easier to achieve and maintain. Consider the polar opposite of a simple meal of baked fish, broccoli, and salad: the 75-item All-You-Can-Eat Buffet! Researchers monitoring buffet eaters have found that diners at all-you-can eat restaurants tend to refill their plates an average of three to five times. (Think about the last time you had a buffet meal. How many times did you refill your dinner plate?) Behavioral studies have shown that the more food options available to a person, the more calories he or she will consume. As

Look Slimmer in 3 Seconds
Take a stand against poor posture.

Got your attention? You can appear trimmer instantly simply by standing up straight. Slouching adds the appearance of extra pounds by forcing your belly to stick out. Stand tall as if there's a string attached to the top of your head pulling you upward. Pull your shoulders back and your belly button in toward your spine. It's no gimmick. This posture engages your core muscles, pulling your belly in and supporting your spine, and instantly makes you look leaner, stronger, and more confident. Plus, this stance allows you to breathe more deeply, which makes you more alert, energized, and youthful.

another example, in one study, subjects were invited to eat from two bowls of M&M candies. Both bowls contained the same number of candies, but one bowl contained more different-colored candies than the other. It turned out that subjects who ate from the bowl containing a greater color variety consumed more of the candy. Researchers say we find variety more appealing, and therefore, we eat more when faced with a greater breadth of food options.

One of the ways you will outsmart that dangerous tendency of human nature is by simplifying your meals on the 7-Day Belly Melt Diet and by sweeping your home of tempting variety, especially if it's in a box, bag, can, or other type of processed-food packaging. See, when you don't have cupcakes on the kitchen counter next to the bowl of apples, you can't be tempted to pass on an apple and go for a cupcake instead.

So let's recap: We're talking about a belly-off plan designed to strip away one to two pounds every single day

Heart Helper
Lose your belly, flex your arteries.

There's no harm in wanting to flatten your belly or fit into skinny jeans, but don't lose sight of a much more important reason to lose weight: to improve heart health. In a study at Johns Hopkins University School of Medicine, researchers studied groups of dieters for six months and found that those who lost the most belly fat also showed an improvement in artery flexibility. Their arteries were able to expand to a greater degree, allowing blood to flow through them more easily. What's more, those dieters who cut calories from carbohydrates and (some but not all) fats lost the most weight and, you guessed it, lost it at a faster pace.

as you do minimal exercise while eating a lot of the foods that you already love.

But wait—what about all those warnings about yo-yo dieting? What about the slowing metabolism and loss of muscle mass that losing weight too fast causes? What about Oprah?

Don't worry. Researchers have figured out how keep your metabolism from getting sleepy and ensure that you stay on the path to leanness for years to come. And believe it or not, part of the answer is to exercise less and eat more.

The 7-Day Belly Melt Diet Difference

Here's why losing weight quickly is the best way to lose weight for good.

SO, JUST WHAT is it about this diet program that allows us to break all the rules and shed pounds so quickly?

Three key principles:

1 Lose weight fast. Dropping significant pounds within a week gives you an incredible boost of confidence in your ability and motivation to stick with your new, healthier lifestyle, even if your weight loss seems to slow down after the pounds initially melt away. In a study by University of Florida researchers, which was published in *the International Journal of Behavioral Medicine,* speedy weight loss showed itself to be more effective than gradual weight loss for the 262 women involved in the trial. Those who lost more than two pounds a week lost more weight overall and better maintained their new bodies compared to the women who lost weight much more gradually. Don't discount the power of motivation. When you lose pounds quickly at the start and then continue to gradually drop weight, you have momentum that helps you maintain the loss.

2 Trim calories without starving. This plan
works by reducing your calorie intake significantly while still keeping your belly full and happy and your metabolism running high. After some initial weight loss, the body's metabolism typically slows down in an attempt to conserve calories. This survival-mode metabolism often frustrates dieters who expect to keep losing fat and pounds at the same rate as they did in the beginning. And their frustration causes them to give up even though they are on the brink of success. This is a critical time in the game. The 7-Day Belly Melt Diet takes this plateau into account and makes certain that levels of the fat-burning hormone *leptin* stay high in the body despite the fact that you are consuming fewer calories and your weight has dropped. You never feel hungry, so you don't reach for high-calorie snacks. And your body never feels as

if it's starving, so it doesn't automatically cannibalize muscle for fuel. Muscle is important for weight maintenance, which we'll get into in more detail later.

3 Target belly fat. As we age, our bodies tend to deposit more fat in our abdomens and thighs. The most worrisome type of fat is the visceral abdominal fat deep in our bellies surrounding our organs because it secretes damaging chemicals and is associated with high cholesterol, high blood pressure, and risk of diabetes and heart disease. The less dangerous fat, the subcutaneous kind just under the skin, is pretty harmless, though some people find it unattractive. It jiggles when you walk. Rapid weight loss can help get rid of both types of fat. In a study in the *International Journal of Obesity and Related Metabolic Disorders*, Finnish researchers found that people who followed an accelerated six-week weight-loss program lost an average of 25 percent visceral belly fat and 16 percent surface or subcutaneous fat. The 7-Day Belly Melt Diet emphasizes fat-burning foods, such as protein and fiber and plant foods rich in a specific kind of nutrient called flavonoids, which influence your cells and keep your body from gaining weight.

The Power of Leptin and Flavonoids

First, let's dig a bit deeper into that fat-burning hormone called leptin (derived from the Greek *leptos* meaning "thin"). The reason most diets fail is that when your body senses that it is taking in fewer calories, it automatically lowers leptin production, reduces metabolism, and stores fat as a conservation measure. See, your body doesn't recognize a dip in calories as something you've planned purposely because you have that date with a pink bikini in two weeks. No, nature takes over and, instinctively, the body's metabolism throttles down to hang onto calories because it perceives a lack of available food and prepares for it to continue for the foreseeable future. Your body's ancient survival instinct doesn't understand that pepperoni pizza can be just a phone call away.

The trick is to keep leptin levels high by tricking your body into feeling that everything is hunky-dory nutrition-wise even while calories are indeed being reduced. You do that by eating meals or snacks at six strategic times of the day (every three hours or so) and by having plenty of specific "high-flavonoid foods" (don't worry; they're delicious), which we'll get to next.

You've probably heard the term *flavonoids,* but you'd be hard-pressed to say exactly what they are or just what they do. In short, they are powerful compounds found in fruits and vegetables that research shows may be one of the most potent weight-loss weapons known to man. Consider this study reported recently in the medical journal *BMJ*. Researchers analyzed lifestyle data about more than 124,000 people middle-aged and older. The scientists noticed that the people who ate diets high in foods containing lots of flavonoids and related compounds—foods like berries, celery, cherries, radishes, peppers, green tea, pears, prunes, and blueberries—either lost weight or maintained their weight better than people who didn't eat such foods or ate little of them. Earlier studies suggest that flavonoids may lower fat absorption and actually boost calorie expenditure.

That's good news for people who like to eat because you can easily add flavonoid-filled foods into your diet without having to give up most of the foods you love. Just remember F.L.A.V.O.R., a simple acronym that we'll explain soon. Setting yourself up for rapid fat loss can be as easy as adding an extra serving of vegetables alongside your barbecued ribs or snacking on an apple after lunch. Each time you eat nutrient-dense F.L.A.V.O.R. foods, you're doing two things: 1. You're filling up on low-calorie, high-volume foods that cause you to automatically eat fewer calorie-dense foods because your hunger is satisfied more quickly. 2. You're accelerating your metabolism with hundreds of different weight-loss compounds, critical nutrients that have been stripped from the American diet by food marketers and packaged-goods manufacturers.

Now, that may all sound well and good, but you no

F.L.A.V.O.R. FOODS

Simplify your diet by focusing on these flavonoid-rich foods that stifle hunger and burn fat.

F reshly Brewed Tea

L entils and Beans

A pples, Berries, and Other Fruits

V egetables and Leafy Greens

O ils, Nuts, and Seeds

R ed Meat and Other Protein Sources

For a full description of the F.L.A.V.O.R. Foods and their health benefits, see Chapter 4, which starts on page 29.

doubt noticed the words "barbecued ribs" up in that last paragraph. It's true; you can eat ribs—and steaks, burgers, bacon, and meatloaf—on this plan. You'll also eat full-fat dairy (even whipped cream) and other fatty foods. You'll eat many different kinds of vegetables and fruits, too. And you'll drink lots of water and tea.

Sounds pretty easy so far, right?

What makes this program all the more exciting is there's no counting calories. There are no special recipes to make (although we've provided a terrific selection for you) and no exotic foods to hunt down. You don't have to tally up points, follow confusing protocols, or order expensive, tasteless, packaged meals to be delivered to your door.

Don't Get Us Wrong about Calories

It's true, you won't have to count calories on the Belly Melt Diet. But that doesn't mean calories don't count. They do! If you want to shed your belly flab, calorie restriction is essential. Anyone who tells you otherwise is blowing smoke. Look, you know you can't eat a half dozen jelly donuts for breakfast and hope to lose weight. It would be ludicrous to think that you could gorge on heaping plates of pasta for dinner and look slim in a bikini in 15 days.

Reducing the number of calories you consume and boosting the number you burn through exercise are absolutely essential if you want to lose your belly rapidly.

Here's proof: In a study published in *The Scandinavian Journal of Medicine & Science in Sports,* 15 healthy but overweight subjects lost 11 pounds (half coming from body fat) in just four days. How did they lose that much so quickly? They consumed just 350 calories per day and they walked for eight hours a day.

Crazy, right? Of course, we're not suggesting anyone go to those extremes to fit into a cocktail dress. But the study demonstrates two important points: 1. how effective the combination of calorie-restriction and exercise can be for quick and dramatic results; and 2. how rapid fat loss can lead to ongoing weight loss. To this second point, the scientists were surprised to learn that most of those people who dropped 11 pounds went on to lose even more weight the by the end of the month and—here's the kicker—they had kept most of the body fat off a year after the experiment ended.

Don't worry: The Belly Melt Diet takes a much more reasonable approach to calorie slash and burn. We know you aren't a test subject with eight hours of free time to stroll through the Scandinavian countryside. We know that you probably have a day job and one at home, too. We want to make healthier eating a no-brainer for you by giving you a simple routine that you can easily follow for *more* than four days.

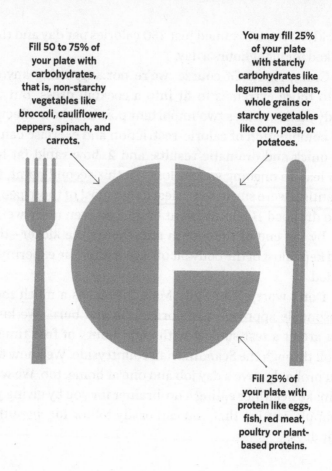

Fill 50 to 75% of your plate with carbohydrates, that is, non-starchy vegetables like broccoli, cauliflower, peppers, spinach, and carrots.

You may fill 25% of your plate with starchy carbohydrates like legumes and beans, whole grains or starchy vegetables like corn, peas, or potatoes.

Fill 25% of your plate with protein like eggs, fish, red meat, poultry or plant-based proteins.

So, here's how we'll put you on reduced-calorie autopilot so you won't even realize it: We want you to think of every meal as though it were a sculpture or a painting—or, if you're more data-driven, as a pie chart like this above.

At every meal, follow the 25/75 rule, roughly 25 percent of your plate will be protein and the remaining 75 percent carbohydrates, mostly vegetables and a small amount of beans or whole grains. For the protein portion, that's a steak, a nice piece of fish, a sizzling burger, some roast beef, a pork chop, a container of Greek yogurt, some tofu—whatever. It will take up 25 percent of your plate. This simple visual cue will give you the proper amount of fat-burning, metabolism-stoking, muscle-strengthening protein you need to stay full and satisfied without overloading you with calories. Protein digests more slowly than carbohydrates do, and has very little impact on your blood sugar. Protein, therefore, is the key to satisfying your hunger. And don't forget, protein builds muscle. Guaranteeing you eat protein at every meal will ensure that your body maintains its muscle even as your body fat begins melting away like Frosty the Snowman in a Bikram yoga class.

The rest of your plate (the remaining 75 percent) will be vegetables and fruits with a little bit of beans, legumes, or whole grains. Now, don't panic: You're not going to be choking down steamed kohlrabi for the next few weeks. You can enjoy your favorite vegetables, whatever they are. Feel free to grill or sauté them in olive oil, or top them with a few pats of butter and some salt if that's how you like them. Extra fat will help your body absorb the flavonoids in the produce, and will keep you full. In fact, the combo of fat and flavonoids is so powerful that we've even created a delicious, creamy, fatty, fruity dessert that you can enjoy each night. (You'll read more about it later.)

This visual approach to proper portion and calorie control requires no math (okay, a little geometry, but no searching to find a food's calorie content or calculating a daily total). Calorie restriction comes naturally and easily through selecting F.L.A.V.O.R. foods and arranging them strategically on your plate.

The 7-Day Belly Melt Die

SIX SIMPLE STEPS

1. Reduce calories and crush hunger by eating six times a day.
2. Eat flavonoid-rich F.L.A.V.O.R. foods.
3. Start your day with a smoothie.
4. Drink more water and unsweetened tea.
5. Do the One Minute Morning Energizer every day.
6. Go to bed earlier. Studies show night owls get fat.

(These steps are explained in detail in Chapter 8.)

Meals

- You will eat six times a day: breakfast, lunch, and dinner, two snacks, and a nightly dessert.

- For breakfast, you'll enjoy a delicious smoothie made to unlock the fat-burning power of protein and flavonoids.

- For lunch and dinner, you'll use the pie chart method. You'll divide your plate into ½ to ¾ non-starchy vegetables and fruits, (on occasion ¼ starchy vegetables, legumes, beans, or whole grains), and ¼ protein: a steak, chicken breast, a bunless burger, a couple of eggs, a cup of yogurt, a pork chop, or a piece of fish. You will top your vegetables with your choice of fats. That could be dressing on a tossed salad, olive oil drizzled over roasted vegetables, a few pats of butter on steamed vegetables, or shredded cheese melting over broccoli.

- You will finish each meal with a serving of fruit, with an emphasis on apples and berries topped with whipped cream. Or you can save dessert for a nighttime snack. Your call.

t a Glance

- Twice a day—whenever you're hungry—you will grab a snack that utilizes the weight-loss powers of fruits and vegetables.

Foods to Focus On

F reshly Brewed Tea

L entils and Beans

A pples, Berries, and Other Fruits

V egetables and Leafy Greens

O ils, Nuts, and Seeds

R ed Meat and Other Protein Sources

Foods to Avoid or Limit

Breads and Cereals

Pastas, Rice, Oats, and Other Grains (limit whole grains and starchy vegetables to ¼ of your plate.)

Added Sugars, Fillers, Additives, and Preservatives

Processed Meats (Sausage, Chicken Nuggets, Deli Meats)

Sweetened Beverages

Alcoholic Beverages

What You'll Drink

Smoothies, teas, water (still or sparkling). You'll drink 16 glasses of cold water a day. Cold water is a calorie-free weight-loss secret weapon. It fills your belly, eliminates false food cravings, improves digestion and energy, and causes your body to burn a few extra calories. Drink up! (And know the location of the closest restroom.)

How You'll Exercise

Each morning before breakfast you'll do our One Minute Morning Energizer. This is just one minute of intense-effort exercise. Don't worry: It's not as daunting as it sounds. You'll break that minute down into 20-second parts interspersed between 90-second recovery periods of easy movement. With a 2-minute warm-up to get the blood flowing, that's just 6 total minutes of your precious morning time and only 1 minute of intense effort.

Now, you might be thinking: *That's crazy. Sixty seconds of exercise and I'll have abs like Jillian Michaels? No way!*

Well, you would be right. Abs in a minute won't happen. You see, countless clinical trials show that a healthier diet that reduces calories is far more effective than exercise for shedding belly fat. That's why you will emphasize food over exercise in the Belly Melt Diet.

But exercise adds a critical ally to your fight against flab: better overall health.

You probably know that the big buzz in fitness is interval-based exercise, also known as high-intensity interval training (or HIIT). Many studies have shown that short bursts of rigorous activity sandwiched in between longer, slower recovery periods burn more calories more efficiently than long, uninterrupted session of slow aerobic activity. And it turns out that the staccato-like interval approach tends to keep your metabolism elevated even after you've stopped exercising—yes, even if you're lounging on a beanbag chair.

Pretty cool, huh?

Now, an interval-exercise workout typically takes 25 minutes or more. Researchers at McMaster University in Canada knew that even 25 minutes is too much for some people to commit to exercise. So they set out to learn how little a person could do while still gaining the health and fitness benefits of longer exercise sessions. The kinesiologists put 14 sedentary and overweight men and women on computerized exercise bicycles. The riders started with 2 minutes of easy pedaling to warm up. Then they were asked to pedal "all-out" (as hard and fast as they could) for 20 seconds then do 2 minutes of slow, easy pedaling to recover. They did this 20-second hard, 2-minutes easy interval twice more. In all, it took 10 minutes, but only 1 minute was intense interval training. The overweight subjects did this workout three times a week. After six weeks, the researchers compared aerobic endurance, blood pressure, and blood sugar levels and found significant improvement in all markers of health and fitness.

So, the point of your One Minute Morning Energizer is NOT to melt your belly. It's the minimum you need to do to guarantee improved health and fitness levels, which will ultimately help you to lose weight. And, by the way, you won't need a stationary bike to do it. We'll show you how to get it done at home, even if you're still in your PJs.

You'll find that your aerobic endurance and energy will improve rapidly, and you'll want to move your body more throughout the day and even tackle some of the longer optional workouts described later in this program.

Back to your biggest weight-loss weapon—food!
Turn the page to see a sample of your daily F.L.A.V.O.R. Foods meal menu.

Sample F.L.A.V.O.R. Foods Menu

Here's what a typical day of eating on The 7-Day Belly Melt Diet looks like:

After your One Minute Morning Energizer:
Drink 16 ounces of ice water (two 8-ounce glasses) with lemon

Breakfast:
Cherry Chocolate Tart Protein Smoothie

Mid-Morning Snack:
Apple with Peanut Butter, 16 ounces of ice water with lemon

Lunch:
Baked Eggs with Mushrooms & Spinach, 16 ounces of ice water

Afternoon Snack:
Carrots and Celery Sticks with Hummus, 16 ounces of ice water

Dinner:
Herb-Roasted Chicken with Root Vegetables, unsweetened iced tea or hot tea, and water.

Dessert:
Mixed Berries with Whipped Cream

- Drink a total of 16 eight-ounce glasses of ice water throughout the day. Don't forget!

Get a
Head Start

No dilly-dallying; let's reap the health benefits of losing weight right away!

THIS SHORT CHAPTER explains exactly how to get going from square one. It'll set you up for success, so don't skip ahead. Whenever you take a journey, you need to know your departure point and your destination. Here's how to begin and what you'll gain from the Belly Melt Diet.

Examine Your Calendar

The first order of business is to circle or highlight the date of whatever event it is that has you hustling to flatten your tummy. Keep that calendar front and center in your life—on your smartphone, stuck to the door of the fridge, on the dashboard of your car. Deadlines motivate people and keep them on track. So use your zero-hour deadline to your advantage.

Weigh Yourself

Hop onto a scale and record your body weight. Depressing? Stop thinking that way. You need a starting point so you have a way of gauging your progress. Several studies have shown that people who weigh themselves regularly are more likely to lose weight and keep it off. It makes sense: Being mindful of your body is an important element in keeping it healthy and fit. Record your starting weight in your journal, another tool you should keep handy. Always weigh yourself at roughly the same time of day for greatest accuracy.

Find Your Waist-to-Hip Ratio

Take a cloth or plastic measuring tape and wrap it around your waist at or just above your belly button. Look in the mirror to make sure the tape is parallel with the floor all the way around. Write down the measurement. Now take a measurement at the widest part of your hips and butt. Write it down. Now divide your waist measurement by your hip measurement to find your waist-to-hip ratio.

Female	Male	
Waist-to-Hip Ratio	**Waist-to-Hip Ratio**	**Health Risk**
0.80 or below	0.95 or below	Low
0.81–0.85	0.96–1.0	Moderate
0.85 or above	1.0 or above	High

That measure is an easy way to very accurately gauge your overall health and the amount of visceral fat you are carrying. Ridding your belly of visceral fat is the key goal of the 7-Day Belly Melt Diet. Re-measure your hip-to-waist every week to see how your belly is shrinking during the initial phase of the program and during the maintenance phase. You may also want to measure each thigh at its thickest part and record those measurements below or in your log, found in the appendix starting on page 163.

In time, you can put down the tape; you'll notice significant fluctuations in your weight and shape simply by the fit of your clothing.

YOUR STARTING MEASUREMENTS

DATE: _____

TIME OF DAY: _____

HEIGHT: _____

WEIGHT: _____

WAIST (Circumference in inches at belly button):

_____

HIPS (Circumference in inches at widest bar of hips):

_____

WAIST-TO-HIP RATIO: _____

LEFT THIGH: _____

RIGHT THIGH: _____

Grab a Tall Glass of Ice Water

Have a seat, and skim the rest of this book or at least re-read the "At a Glance" section. You'll want to get the lay of the land before diving right in. And the emphasis on water? We want you to get in the habit of drinking a lot more water every day, so start right now with some ice water or hot water with a spritz of lemon. There are a couple of reasons for this. One, water takes up room in your belly, making you feel less hunger. That's why you should always begin a meal by drinking a glass of water or a cup of broth. Penn State nutritionist Barbara Rolls, PhD, says foods with a naturally high water content generally have low energy densities, meaning they fill you up without loading you up with calories. In one of her studies, participants were served a chicken casserole or chicken and rice soup. It turned out that the soup eaters consumed 26 percent less than the casserole eaters. Water also helps your body digest food properly and absorb vitamins and nutrients from the food. You won't get enough from eating low-water-content foods or even drinking water with dinner. You need to make a conscious effort to drink more water throughout the day. Keep a water bottle filled with ice water, and bring it with you wherever you go.

Track Your Meals and Beverages

Use the Food & Fitness Tracker in the appendix to record what you eat and drink. Remember, you don't have to count calories on this program. But the simple act of writing down what you have eaten every day is a powerful habit to get into. By doing so, you're learning to be mindful of what you eat. The act reinforces the principles of the Belly Melt Diet and helps you ensure you're loading up on F.L.A.V.O.R. foods.

Snap a Photo

Take a snapshot of yourself wearing a bathing suit. A selfie will work, but for a better image, ask a friend or your spouse to take two digital shots of you: one facing forward and one from the side. No sucking in that belly! Let it all hang out. This is another useful tool to remind you of your goal, and to measure your progress through comparison.

Make a Confession

Finally, tell a friend what you're doing or post it on social media. Better yet, recruit a compadre to join you on your speedy flat-belly quest. You're more likely to stick with a program and find success if you make your plans public and if a friend joins you on the journey.

Sign a Contract

Make a promise to yourself that you will give the Belly Melt Diet your best effort. (See page 20.) Also, promise yourself that you will not beat yourself up if you don't follow your plan to a T. Often, giving yourself a Mulligan, to use a golf term, is all you need to get back on track. And think about it—the world's tough enough on you; you don't need to pile on. Fall down. Get up. Give yourself a hug. Move forward. Got it?

The 7-Day Belly Melt Diet Contract

I promise myself that I will do everything in my power to follow the F.L.A.V.O.R. Meal Plan, do my One Minute Morning Energizer each morning, drink 16 glasses of water every day, and avoid processed foods and fast-burning carbohydrates throughout the 7-Day Belly Melt Diet. I will complete this program to establish healthy eating habits for life—and look leaner, fitter, and healthier by (DATE:_____).

_____   _____
SIGNED   DATE

Benefits to Expect from the 7-Day Belly Melt Diet

There are a lot of ways to lose weight. There are a lot of ways to lose weight fast. But there aren't a lot of ways to lose weight rapidly, safely, and forever while also putting yourself on the path to better long-term health and a fitter, stronger body. The 7-Day Belly Melt Diet delivers these important health benefits:

- **You'll maintain your weight loss for decades to come.** Three cohort studies monitoring nearly 125,000 people for 24 years published in *BMJ* found that the people who ate the most flavonoids were the most successful in keeping their weight under control. The most powerful foods included blueberries, apples, pears, prunes, strawberries, grapes, peppers, celery, and green tea.

- **You'll protect your heart.** A study of nearly 35,000 women over 16 years found that those with the highest intake of flavonoids—in particular anthocyanidins, flavones, and flavanones—had the lowest incidence of cardiovascular disease. Apples, pears, red wine, grapefruit, strawberries, and dark chocolate seemed to have the most noticeable effect.

- **You'll dodge the dangers of diabetes.** High levels of flavonoids—especially those found in chocolate, tea, and berries—seem to help regulate blood glucose, according to a 2014 study published in the *Journal of Nutrition*. The study focused on two types of flavonoids: flavones, which are found in vegetables like celery and herbs like thyme and parsley, and anthocyanins, which lend red and blue color to berries, red grapes, and wine. In the study, those who consumed the most flavone compounds had higher levels of a protein called adiponectin, which has been shown to battle belly fat in particular.

- **You'll bring down high blood pressure if you have hypertension.** Over a two-week period, daily small doses of flavonoid-rich dark chocolate improved the ability of subjects' blood vessels to dilate, reducing the risk of stroke and heart disease, according to a study in the *Journal of the American College of Nutrition*.

Subjects who got high-quality dark chocolate showed an increase in arterial flexibility, while control subjects who got lesser, flavonoid-poor chocolate actually saw their arteries stiffen more, researchers found. (To make sure you're getting the benefits, look for a label indicating it's 70 percent cacao or higher.)

- **You'll reduce your risk of inflammatory diseases.** Atherosclerosis and a myriad of other diseases, from obesity to allergies to inflammatory bowel disease to psoriasis and certain forms of arthritis, are linked to the inflammatory response in our bodies. A 2014 study in the *European Journal of Medicinal Chemistry* found that flavonoids inhibit a compound called lipoxygenase, or LOX, that facilitates the spread of inflammation throughout the body.

- **You'll protect yourself from Parkinson's disease.** Researchers at the University of East Anglia reported that flavonoid-rich foods including berries, apples, and red wine significantly reduce the risk of developing Parkinson's. The study, published in the journal *Neurology*, looked at 130,000 men and women and found that, in the men at least, those who ate the most flavonoids were 40 percent less likely to develop the disease than those who ate the least. In fact, just one serving of berries a week reduced their risk of Parkinson's by 25 percent.

- **Your brain will stay younger longer.** A 2012 study found that elderly women who consumed a lot of blueberries and strawberries delayed their cognitive aging by up to two-and-a-half years compared to the women who consumed the least of these flavonoid-rich berries. The study, published in *Annals of Neurology*, focused on data from more than 16,000 women over the age of 70. Over the course of six years, the berry eaters showed significantly better memory and cognitive function than those who ate less.

  By stripping away belly fat, flavonoids will help protect your brain in other ways. For years, scientists have understood that midlife obesity is a risk factor for dementia later in life. Just as belly fat helps cause the formation of plaque in your coronary arteries, so too does it clog up the arteries that feed the brain—a contributing factor in the development of Alzheimer's. According to research at

Rush University Medical Center, the protein responsible for metabolizing fat in the liver is the same protein found in the hippo-campus, the part of the brain that controls memory and learning. People with higher levels of abdominal fat actually have depleted levels of this fat-metabolizing protein, making them 3.6 times more likely to suffer from memory loss and dementia later in life.

But a few years ago, scientists discovered something even more ominous. They performed CT scans on a number of healthy middle-aged men and women to measure their visceral fat. What they learned was that the more visceral fat a person had, the less brain mass he or she had.

- **You'll put more money in your pocket.** Consider this: Obese women fork over an additional $8,365 every year in health-care costs (doctor visits, over-the-counter and prescription medicines, and the like) than healthy-weight women. In fact, by one estimate, obesity-related health care will cost Americans $190 billion during this year alone.

  But the real cost of being overweight doesn't come in the form of prescription pills and diet products. It's not the money we spend; it's the money we don't make. In a study published in the *International Journal of Obesity*, researchers gave participants a series of résumés with small photos of the applicants attached. What they learned was that starting salary, leadership potential, and hiring decisions were all negatively impacted when the photo showed a person who was overweight—most severely in the case of obese women. One study by researchers at the University of Florida found that the thinnest women made a whopping $22,283 more than their overweight peers. That means that for American women, gaining 25 pounds results in an average salary loss of $15,572.

  Think of it this way: An overweight woman who works for 25 years will wind up with $389,300 less than a thinner one. Add in 25 years of paying that extra eight grand in health-care costs, and the total swing between slender and stocky amounts to $598,425.

- **You'll improve your love life.** In studies, women with excess abdominal fat have been shown to have elevated secretions of cortisol, a stress hormone, and an increased sensitivity to stress hormones in the hypothalamus, pituitary, and adrenal glands. Cortisol makes us gain belly fat, so more belly fat equals more cortisol, which equals more belly fat, a nasty cycle. But worse, women who show an increase in cortisol in response to sexual stimuli have lower levels of functioning in certain areas of their sex life compared with women who show a decrease in cortisol. Good sex comes from less stress. Abdominal fat causes more stress, which causes bad sex. You get the picture.

- **You'll feel happier!** Folate, a B vitamin that rides along with flavonoids in green vegetables and legumes, is something of a miracle drug when it comes to managing your mood. Low levels of folate have been linked to depression, low energy levels, and even memory loss, and studies show that adding folate-rich foods like green tea, beans, and lettuces reduces fatigue, improves energy levels, and helps battle depression. And new research published in the British journal *Age and Ageing* indicates that losing belly fat may be the most significant thing you can do to improve your life as you get older. In a study, researchers surveyed nearly 600 men between the ages of 60 and 74, asking them about a wide range of issues, from their physical health to their social lives to their mental and emotional well-being. What they discovered was that the greatest single factor impacting quality of life was belly fat—the more belly fat these men had, the more likely they were to report unhappiness with their lives.

The Flavonoid Advantage

It pays to eat a more colorful diet.

FLAVONOID—IT DOESN'T exactly roll off the tongue. Spoken softly, the term might be confused for an inflammatory condition you'd remedy with a tube of Preparation H. But make no mistake, unlike hemorrhoids, you don't want to get rid of flavonoids; you want more of them.

Flavonoids could easily be called Polaroids, because their most obvious function is to give color to plants: the deep purples of winter kale, the verdant greens of spring lettuces, the mellow yellows of summer squash, the rich ambers of autumn's pumpkins, and the fire-engine red of chile peppers all come from flavonoids. One of flavonoids' main functions is to attract bees, butterflies, and other pollinators to the plant to ensure it continues into the next generation. They also help inhibit certain diseases that can sap a plant's energy.

When abundant in our diets, flavonoids become nutritional superstars capable of all sorts of medical miracles. The flavonoid class of beneficial compounds includes catechins, polyphenols, anthoxanthins, anthocyanins, and other various terms that look kind of like flavonoid, such as flavones and flavan-3-ols. While flavonoids have been shown to help battle everything from cancer to allergies, their greatest power is as an anti-inflammatory. By reducing the levels of inflammation in the body, they provide powerful protection against disease while turning your body's weight-loss switches to "on."

You don't need to remember the names of all these flavonoid compounds. Just eat a broad variety of fruits and vegetables during the course of a week and you'll be guaranteed to consume the following categories, which are the most beneficial.

The Belly Melters: Anthocyanidins

WHAT THEY DO: Help battle obesity, diabetes, cancer, heart disease, and inflammation.

WHERE TO FIND THEM: There are more than 635 versions of these compounds (they're known as anthocyanins when they're joined with sugar molecules); they're responsible for the coloring of most fruits, but they're hard to find in vegetables; only red potatoes, red onions, and red cabbage, as well as beans, eggplant, and chard, have significant levels.

WHAT YOU NEED TO KNOW: Eat plenty of fruit and you should get all the anthocyanidins you need, but be wary if you live north of, say, Baltimore: A 2011 study of European food habits in the *British Journal of Nutrition* found that the farther north people live, the lower their intake of anthocyanidins is likely to be. People in southern Italy eat more than three times as many as people in The Netherlands.

The Heart Helpers: Flavan-3-ols

WHAT THEY DO: Improve arterial flow, reduce blood pressure, and help prevent heart disease and diabetes. In a 2012 review of 42 studies, researchers reporting in the *American Journal of Clinical Nutrition* found consistent evidence that flavan-3-ols improved cardiovascular health and reduced diabetes risk. They also have antiviral and cancer-fighting properties.

WHERE TO FIND THEM: Flavan-3-ols impart a bitter taste, which explains why they're found not just in berries and tree fruits, but also in high concentrations in dark chocolate, dark beer, tea, and coffee. Among vegetables, only legumes deliver these nutrients.

WHAT YOU NEED TO KNOW: Processing destroys flavan-3-ols, so if you're eating Dutch or alkalized chocolate, you're probably not getting much at all. Make sure your chocolate has 70 percent cacao or better. To muscle up your coffee, order an Americano instead of a traditional drip coffee; it's made with espresso, which is higher in flavan-3-ols than regular brewed coffee.

The Energizers: Flavonols

WHAT THEY DO: May improve both mental and physical performance on tests by boosting overall endurance. They've also been shown to reduce cholesterol and C-reactive protein (CRP), a marker of inflammation. In a 2012 analysis of studies, men and women with the highest intake of these nutrients had an 18 percent lower risk of heart disease; other studies suggest that flavonols reduce stroke risk by 20 percent.

WHERE TO FIND THEM: Flavonols are pale yellow in color, and are found in a wide variety of vegetables, including leafy greens, onions, tea, chia seeds, and buckwheat, and in the skins of fruits like apples, cherry tomatoes, pears, and berries.

WHAT YOU NEED TO KNOW: It makes sense to eat seasonally: During summer months, leafy greens like lettuce and leeks have been found to have three to five times more flavonols than in other seasons.

The Age Erasers: Flavones

WHAT THEY DO: Prevent oxidative stress—what we call aging. They've also been shown to help protect against stress-related diseases, including heart disease, diabetes, and cognitive decline, according to a 2014 review in *Current Topic Medical Chemistry.*

WHERE TO FIND THEM: A wide variety of fruits, especially watermelon, contain them, as do tea, coffee, and chocolate; cruciferous vegetables like iceberg lettuce, cauliflower, Brussels sprouts, and cabbage; and leafy greens like mint, parsley, and celery. Also found in hot peppers.

WHAT YOU NEED TO KNOW: Flavones help control histamine, the chemical released during allergic reactions, and can reduce the effects of asthma and allergies.

The Fat Burners: Flavonones

WHAT THEY DO: Reduce stroke risk and strengthen brain function, reduce appetite and increase weight loss.

WHERE TO FIND THEM: Flavonones aren't found in any vegetables at all. You'll get them mostly from citrus fruits like grapefruit, oranges, lemons, and limes. Peppermint leaves have them, too.

WHAT YOU NEED TO KNOW: Daily intake of citrus fruits has been linked to weight loss in several studies; research into the role flavonones play in the belly-flattening powers of citrus is ongoing. A study at the University of Western Ontario in 2009, published in the journal *Diabetes,* found that a particular flavonoid found in citrus, called naringenin, genetically reprograms the liver to burn up excess fat, rather than store it—in the process lowering cholesterol levels and preventing the development of insulin resistance.

The F.L.A.V.O.R. Foods and How They Work

Make losing pounds automatic by filling your plate with these delicious and satisfying superfoods.

YOU CAN JUDGE the effectiveness of any diet by walking into a deli and asking yourself one question: Do I know what to eat?

If you can't glance at a menu board and instantly identify the foods that fit into your plan, then your plan isn't going to hold up in the long run. That's because our brains run on glucose—blood sugar, the same stuff that fuels our muscles and keeps every element of our bodies running efficiently. When you're hungry, your brain functions just a little bit less effectively, and so making smart choices can be more difficult. If your diet requires any sort of mathematical calculation, such as counting calories or points, or prohibits *too many* types of foods, eventually your brain is just going to conk out on you, and you're certain to find yourself pointing to the nearest source of greasy, juicy calories and saying, "I'll take two."

That's why having an easy-to-remember guide is so important. So to keep you fit, focused, and full, we created the F.L.A.V.O.R. system.

F reshly Brewed Tea

L entils and Beans

A pples, Berries, and Other Fruits

V egetables and Leafy Greens

O ils, Nuts, and Seeds

R ed Meat and Other Protein Sources

The acronym helps you recall these foods that are always available, always satisfying. It will help you develop a habit of eating mostly whole foods, that is, foods that are as close as possible to what's available in nature. Doing so automatically reduces calories and eliminates the inflammatory ingredients found in processed foods. And each of these F.L.A.V.O.R. food groups has its own remarkable powers that will help you banish your belly with shocking speed.

FRESHLY BREWED TEA

Think of your body as a teapot on the stove, and think of the water inside of it as your belly fat. Chances are the pot is sitting there over a low flame, not doing much of anything. The water inside might be warm, but it's not boiling away. If you want the teapot to whistle—and attract a few whistles of your own—you need to crank up the heat.

Well, that's what tea—and specifically, freshly brewed tea—will do for you. You see, bottled teas (the Snapples of the world) are often loaded with natural or artificial sweeteners, which pack on pounds even as they damage our ever-so-valuable belly biomes. And more important, the longer a tea sits around in a bottle, the more the flavonoids inside it begin to break down. A few years back, the authors of *Eat This, Not That!* commissioned a study of bottled green teas and found that store-bought teas typically lose about 20 percent of their flavonoid content during the bottling process. And as time goes by, and the tea is exposed to light and heat, the powerful weight-loss compounds erode even further: More than 50 percent of the flavonoids are gone within three months.

By contrast, when you brew your own tea, you unleash a flavonoid bounty that will take direct aim at your belly fat. And because there are so many different types of teas—each with their own fat-burning powers—you can experiment and constantly keep your palate, and your body, guessing. Here are some of the teas you should work into your day. The more tea you drink, the greater your flavonoid intake— and the faster your weight loss.

Green Tea: Green tea is particularly high in a type of flavonoid called EGCG, which can "turn off" the genetic triggers for obesity and diabetes. EGCG also boosts levels of a hunger-quelling hormone called cholecystokinin. In one Swedish study, people who sipped green tea reported less of a desire to eat their favorite foods even two hours after drinking the brew. And people who consume at least

120 milliliters of green tea—that's about half a cup—each day for a year have a 46 percent lower risk of developing hypertension than those who consume less, according to a study in the *Archives of Internal Medicine*. In another study, people who combined a daily habit of four to five cups of green tea with a 25-minute daily workout lost an average of two pounds more during a 12-week study than exercisers who didn't sip the tea. What makes the drink so powerful? It contains catechins, flavonoids that hinder the storage of belly fat and aid rapid weight loss.

White Tea: A study published in the *Journal of Nutrition and Metabolism* showed that white tea can simultaneously boost lipolysis (the breakdown of fat) and block adipogenesis (the formation of new fat cells) thanks to its high levels of catechins. And a study from Case Western Reserve University found that chemicals in white tea appear to protect skin from sun-induced stress, preventing premature aging.

Black Tea: During times of stress, your body manufactures cortisol, a hormone that gathers up fatty acids in the bloodstream and stores them in your belly. Black tea can help reduce cortisol levels, preventing stress from causing the fat-storage stress reaction. Drinking 20 ounces of black tea daily causes the body to secrete five times as much interferon, a key element in your body's infection-protection arsenal.

Oolong Tea: Otherwise known as "black dragon," oolong tea contains flavonoids that help promote weight loss by boosting your body's ability to metabolize fat. A study in the *Chinese Journal of Integrative Medicine* found that participants who regularly sipped oolong tea lost six pounds over the course of a six-week time period.

Red Tea: South African researchers report that red tea, also known as rooibos, contains flavonoids (in particular a unique flavonoid called aspalathin) that can inhibit the formation of new fat cells by as much as 22 percent. Aspalathin can also reduce stress hormones that trigger hunger and fat storage and reduce the risk of hypertension, metabolic syndrome, cardiovascular disease, and diabetes.

Herbal Teas: Certain herbal teas not only help to soothe the nerves and set the tone for a relaxed evening, but many also have high levels of fat-melting flavonoids. Barberry tea, for instance, can help boost metabolism and reduce fat storage; goji tea has been shown to crank up calorie burn by as much as 10 percent; and numerous studies have shown that flavonoids found in hibiscus tea help to flatten your belly by regulating the hormones that affect your body's electrolyte balance and fluid retention.

LENTILS AND BEANS

Every lentil or bean is like a little weight-loss pill. Legumes (a term for any food that grows in a pod, like lentils, beans, peanuts, and peas) are rich in resistant starch, which has very minimal impact on your blood sugar levels as it passes through the body undigested like fiber. One study found that people who ate ¾ cup of beans daily weighed 6.6 pounds less than those who didn't—even though the bean eaters consumed, on average, 199 more calories per day.

Beans may be the most powerful diabetes-fighting medicine in the grocery store. In one study, diabetics who ate a one-cup serving of beans every day for three months saw better improvements in their blood sugar levels and body weight than those who ate other sources of fiber. And a longer study that followed 64,000 women for an average of 4.6 years found that a high intake of beans was associated with a 38 percent reduced risk for diabetes. But of all the beans in the grocery store, kidney beans pack the biggest dietary fiber wallop; just ½ cup of kidney beans provides 14 grams—more than in three servings of oatmeal! It's not just run-of-the-mill fiber, but that special resistant starch we mentioned earlier. This type of carbohydrate takes longer to digest than others, making it a "low-glycemic" carb, so it helps prevent blood sugar spikes. If you typically buy canned beans, check the label for additives like sugar and salt and rinse your beans thoroughly before digging in.

There's another kind of bean worth mentioning here: the cocoa bean. We don't usually think of chocolate as coming from beans, but it does, and the more of that bean you can get into your diet, the better. University of California–San Diego researchers found that adults who regularly eat chocolate are actually thinner than those who eat chocolate less often, regardless of exercise or calorie intake. Researchers say the belly-slimming properties of chocolate are unlocked in our gut, where good bacteria ferment the cocoa into anti-inflammatory compounds that can "turn off" genes that are linked to obesity.

The flavonoids in chocolate can also lower blood pressure, improve your cholesterol profile, and lower your risk of heart attack by up to 31 percent, according to studies published in the journals *Age* and *the British Journal of Nutrition*. Other scientific findings indicate that cocoa's flavanols can help the body form nitrites, the same chemical in beets and beet greens that widens blood vessels, eases blood flow, and lowers blood pressure levels. The secret is to eat the right kind of chocolate. Most commercial chocolates are processed in ways that destroy many of the nutrients. Make sure your bar has at least 70 percent cacao (the flavonoid-rich cocoa bean), although more is better. We like Alter Eco Blackout and Green & Black's Organic 85 percent Cacao Bar.

APPLES, BERRIES, AND OTHER FRUITS

Because fruit is high in a form of natural sugar called fructose, many diets—especially traditional "low-carb" diets—limit fruits, with some practically banning them entirely. But cutting fruit out of your diet may be one of the worst things you can do if you're looking to achieve both rapid and long-term weight loss. It's one of those simplistic approaches to weight loss—right up there with "don't eat fat"—that got us into this whole obesity crisis in the first place.

That's because, with the exception of a very small handful of purplish vegetables (eggplant, red onion, blue and red potatoes, and black beans), fruits are the only place you'll find the powerful weight-loss compounds called anthocyanidins (or anthocyanins, as they're often called, especially when combined with the natural sugars in fruit). A *Journal of Agricultural and Food Chemistry* study found that anthocyanins could reduce insulin production by as much as 50 percent, which means less fat storage and a reduced risk of diabetes. The deeper the fruit's color, the greater its level of anthocyanins. That means Pink Lady over Granny Smith, watermelon over honeydew, red grapes over green ones. Higher levels of flavonoids—particularly anthocyanins, compounds that give red fruits their color— calm the action of fat-storage genes. In fact, red-bellied stone fruits like plums boast phenolic compounds that have been shown to modulate the expression of fat genes.

The deep color of berries is a signal that they're one of the very best fatburners known to man. Not only are they loaded with flavonoids, but they also actively burn belly fat, practically spot-reducing it! A University of Michigan study found that rats that ate blueberry powder as part of their meals lost belly fat and had lower cholesterol, even when they ate a high-fat diet. It's theorized that the flavonoids in blueberries activate the fat-burning gene in bellyfat cells. Researchers at Tufts University found that people who regularly consumed berry-based flavonoids increased their belly-fat loss by 77 percent.

Additionally, blueberries may be muscle builders. Their skins are rich in ursolic acid, a chemical that a study at the University of Iowa found prevents muscle breakdown in lab animals. According to an *Annals of Neurology* report, consuming a diet rich in blueberries and strawberries may help slow mental decline and help you maintain memory and focus into your golden years. Strawberries are also rich in folate, a nutrient that when it's consumed with B vitamins has been shown to prevent cognitive decline and dementia.

But as you read earlier in this book, a variety of fruits means a variety of flavonoids: No one fruit contains all five categories, regardless of its color. That's why citrus, with its unique flavonoid compounds, is so important. For example, a study in the journal *Metabolism* found that eating half a grapefruit before meals may help reduce visceral fat and lower cholesterol levels. Participants in the six-week study who ate a Rio Red grapefruit 15 minutes before breakfast, lunch, and dinner saw their waists shrink by up to an inch and their LDL levels drop by 18 points. Researchers attribute the effects to a combination of flavonoids and vitamin C in the grapefruit. Consider slicing a few segments for a starter salad, or eating one for a snack shortly before a meal.

VEGETABLES AND LEAFY GREENS

We're not going to shock you by telling you to eat more vegetables. Like saving for retirement and quitting smoking, it's one of those boring-but-obvious good-for-you moves that nobody's going to disagree with. But how much should you eat, and what types? The answer's simple: Eat as much as you can of whatever you can get your hands on. Unless it's covered with breadcrumbs and fried in unhealthy oils (a bit more about that later in this chapter), a vegetable is your friend. The same rules that apply to fruits also apply to vegetables: The deeper the color, the more flavonoids.

Dark leafy greens. You already know that broccoli, kale, and spinach are the Batman, Superman, and Wonder Woman of nutrition. Packed with vitamins, minerals, and fiber. they're also rich in sulforaphane, a compound that blocks enzymes linked to joint destruction and inflammation. But other less-common greens deserve a spot on your plate, too.

Romaine lettuce. Even more so than its cousin kale, humble Romaine packs high levels of folic acid, a water-soluble form of vitamin B that's proven to boost male fertility, battle depression, and help reduce fat storage.

Parsley. Yes, that leafy garnish that sits on the side of your plate—the one restaurants throw away after you eat the rest of your meal—is a quiet superfood, so packed with nutrients that even that one sprig can go a long way toward meeting your daily requirement for vitamin K. Moreover, research suggests the summery aroma and flavor of chopped parsley may help control your appetite. A study in the journal *Flavour* found participants ate significantly less of a dish that smelled strongly of spice than a mildly scented version of the same food. Adding herbs like parsley creates the sensory illusion that you're indulging in something rich—without adding any fat or calories to your plate.

Collard greens. A staple vegetable of Southern U.S. cuisine, collard greens also boast incredible cholesterol-lowering benefits—especially when steamed. A recent study published in the journal *Nutrition Research* compared the effectiveness of the prescription drug Cholestyramine with that of steamed collards. Incredibly, the collards improved the body's cholesterol-blocking process 13 percent better than the drug did!

Chard. Sounds like what you'd say when you've overcooked your burger. It's not as fun a name to drop as, say, "broccolini," but it might be your best defense against diabetes. Recent research has shown that these powerhouse leaves contain at least 13 different polyphenol antioxidants, including anthocyanins, anti-inflammatory compounds that could offer protection from type 2 diabetes. Researchers from the University of East Anglia analyzed questionnaires and blood samples of about 2,000 people and found that those with the highest dietary intakes of anthocyanins had lower insulin resistance and better blood glucose regulation.

Chinese cabbage. In a study of more than 1,000 Chinese women, published in the *Journal of the Academy of Nutrition and Dietetics*, those who ate the most cruciferous vegetables (about 1.5 cups per day) had 13 percent less obesity-causing inflammation than those who ate the least.

Watercress. Gram for gram, this mild-tasting and flowery-looking green contains four times more beta-carotene than an apple, along with a whopping 238 percent of your daily recommended intake of vitamin K per 100 grams—two compounds that keep skin dewy and youthful. The beauty food is also the richest source of a flavonoid called PEITC (phenylethyl isothiocyanate), which research suggests can fight cancer. Results from an eight-week trial published in the *American Journal of Clinical Nutrition* suggest daily supplementation of about two cups of raw watercress could reduce DNA damage by 17 percent.

Orange vegetables. Thanks to their vitamin A and betacarotene content, vegetables like orange peppers and carrots are strong inflammation fighters. These sunny-colored veggies are also rich in betacryptoxanthin, a type of carotenoid pigment that may ward off arthritis.

Purple vegetables. As you've already read, purple signals the presence of anthocyanins—common among fruits but rare among veggies. One of the vegetables rich in this type of flavonoid is eggplant. The shiny purple veggie does more than just help with weight loss; its anthocyanins also provide neuroprotective benefits like bolstering short-term memory. Several studies have found that anthocyanins can help prevent heart disease, too, by reducing inflammation and decreasing arterial hardening.

Red vegetables. Bright-red vegetables like tomatoes and peppers are packed with vitamins A and C and the critical flavonoid quercetin, a powerful antihistamine and antioxidant. They also pack chalconaringenin, kaempferol -3-rutinoside, and myriad other important flavonoids, as well as the cancer-fighting nutrient lycopene.

OILS, NUTS, AND SEEDS

No aspect of nutrition is more confusing than fats and oils. Polyunsaturated, monounsaturated, saturated, trans fats, omega-3s, omega-6s—which ones are good for you again? Actually, the answer to that question depends on who is answering. A lot of well-meaning doctors—including those at the USDA—will tell you to cut down on saturated fat and concentrate on unsaturated fat. Saturated fats come mainly from such animal sources as butter, cheese, milk, beef, poultry, pork, and lamb. The American Heart Association also recommends limiting saturated fats because they raise the level of cholesterol in your blood. But that wisdom started to be questioned several years ago when a meta-analysis of 21 studies found that there was not enough evidence to conclude that saturated fat increases heart disease risk. Highly processed carbohydrates came to replace saturated fats as the heart disease culprit. Medium-chain triglycerides like the saturated fats in coconut oil became popular because they increase leptin, which reduces appetite and makes you feel full, and they are less likely to be stored as body fat. What's more, studies showed that the most common form of polyunsaturated fat, soybean oil, might be as bad for you as just about any food under the sun.

When it comes to oils, most kinds are good for you, especially the monounsaturated kind in olive and canola oils, avocados, and nuts and seeds, as well as in foods made from these sources: peanut and almond butter, guacamole, and olive oil–based dressings. Walnuts, in particular, are a nutritional bonus: Not only are they one of the best dietary sources of monounsaturated fats, but they're also a top source of omega-3 fatty acids, which have been shown to improve brain function. And in a recent study, researchers found that cooking vegetables in olive oil actually increased their levels of flavonoids; the oil is so rich in the good stuff that its flavonoids get transferred into the foods that are fried in it.

Unfortunately, most of the oils we eat come from one source: soybean oil. It's the primary ingredient in most vegetable oils, which means it's a major ingredient in just about every fried, baked, or sautéed food you eat. In a review in the journal *Nutrition,* researchers reported that the type of polyunsaturated fat in soybean oil has been shown to be adipogenic, meaning that it promotes fat storage in our bodies. It also spurs inflammation, and it causes your fat cells to swell in order to retain more fatty acids.

Soybean oil—and its cousins corn oil, safflower oil, and sunflower oil—even seems to mess up our hormonal response to food, increasing our levels of ghrelin (the "I'm hungry" hormone) and reducing our levels of leptin (the "no thanks, I'm full" hormone). In fact, soybean oil may be a more potent cause of obesity than even sugar itself. A recent study at the University of California–Riverside found that, in mice at least, a diet high in soybean oil causes more obesity and diabetes than a diet high in sugar.

Nuts and seeds make the list of F.L.A.V.O.R. foods for their amazing ability to crush hunger pangs. While they are high in calories, they are also rich in satiating protein, fiber, and healthy fats, so you need only a handful as a hunger-busting snack. Raw, unsalted almonds are a particularly powerful snack food. Think of each almond as a natural weight-loss pill. A study of overweight and obese adults found that, combined with a calorie-restricted diet, consuming a little more than a quarter cup of the nuts could decrease weight more effectively than a snack made up of complex carbohydrates and safflower oil—after just two weeks! (And after 24 weeks, those who ate the nuts experienced a 62 percent greater reduction in weight and BMI!) For optimal results, eat your daily serving before you hit the gym: A study printed in *The Journal of the International Society of Sports Nutrition* found that almonds, rich in the amino acid L-arginine, can help you burn more fat and carbs during workouts.

If you get tired of almonds, try flavorful pistachios as a weight-loss snack. Consider the results of this study in which UCLA Center for Human Nutrition researchers divided study participants into two groups, feeding each a nearly identical low-calorie diet for 12 weeks. The only difference between what the groups ate was in what they were given as an afternoon snack. One group ate 220 calories of pretzels, while the other group munched on 240 calories of pistachios. Just four weeks into the study, members of the pistachio group had reduced their body mass index (BMI) by a point, while the BMIs of the pretzel-eating group stayed the same. The pistachio eaters' cholesterol and triglyceride levels showed improvements, as well.

RED MEAT AND OTHER PROTEIN SOURCES

Whether or not you subsist on a ribs-and-burgers diet or live a vegan lifestyle and carefully balance your vegetable proteins, chances are you need more of this essential muscle food, especially if you want rapid weight loss.

Consider this: The Recommended Daily Allowance (RDA) for men is 56 grams of protein a day, while for women it's 46 grams. That's about as much as you'd get in four to five chicken drumsticks or two large hamburgers. Other ways to get close to those numbers: 2½ pork chops, 15 slices of bacon, or an 8-ounce steak.

But that's still not enough: In a 2015 study in the *American Journal of Physiology—Endocrinology and Metabolism,* researchers found that those who ate twice as much protein as the RDA had greater net protein balance and muscle protein synthesis—in other words, it was easier for them to maintain and build muscle, and hence keep their metabolisms revving on high. So even if you eat a burger for lunch and a couple of pork chops for dinner, you're still coming up short in the protein department.

In fact, one of the biggest dietary issues Americans tend

to face is an imbalance in our protein intake. We eat plenty at dinner, but typical breakfasts and lunches are often lacking. That's why the Belly Melt Diet ensures that you'll be getting a hefty dose of protein at every meal.

The Ultimate Flavonoid Fruit Salad

Get one serving a day from each of these four groups.

Many fruits contain solid combinations of the flavonoids: Tree fruits like apples, pears, and cherries deliver three of the five major categories, as do dark red and purple berries like cranberries, blueberries, strawberries, and raspberries. But no fruit delivers all five, which is why mixing it up is so important. In other words, just piling up the apples every day won't keep the doctor away. To make it simple, follow this handy chart. Get a big bowl and mix in one fruit from each of these five beneficial buckets.

THE TREE GROUP

High in anthocyanidins, flavan-3-ols, flavones, and flavonols

- **Apples (with the skin on)**
- **Pears**
- **Cherries**
- **Peaches**
- **Plums**

THE BERRY GROUP

High in anthocyanidins, flavan-3ols, flavones, and flavonols

- **Blackberries**
- **Blueberries**
- **Cranberries**
- **Elderberries**
- **Raspberries**
- **Strawberries**

THE CITRUS GROUP

High in flavones and flavonones

- **Blood oranges**
- **Grapefruit (white or pink)**
- **Lemons**
- **Limes**
- **Oranges**
- **Tangelos**
- **Tangerines**

THE WILDCARD GROUP

High in flavones and a variety of other flavonoids

- **Apricots**
- **Currants**
- **Grapes**
- **Kiwi**
- **Watermelon**

The Exercise Paradox

Get more fitness benefits
from less exercise.

H

AVE YOU EVER WATCHED a baseball or football game and been surprised by the size of the men on the field? Not their muscles—their bellies. Baseball stars have plenty of girth to put behind their swing, even though they're doing daily workouts from April through October. And on the gridiron, nearly half a dozen current NFL players exceed the 350-pound mark, with physiques that jiggle as much as they juke—despite twice-a-day workouts on the field and in the gym.

While consuming mass quantities is no doubt part of these behemoths' secret, it's sometimes hard to believe that men who exercise so much, day in and day out, and whose livelihoods depend on their being as fast and fit as possible, can be so heavy. How is it possible that they can burn off hundreds, perhaps thousands, of extra calories every day and still be so roly-poly?

You probably see the same thing—albeit on a smaller scale—in your gym, or on the jogging path near your office, or on the bike paths during the weekends. People who are exercising hard—sometime even training for marathons or triathlons—but whose bodies seem utterly insistent on holding on to every single fat cell.

There's a reason for that, and in 2015 the *British Journal of Sports Medicine* summed it up nicely: "You cannot outrun a bad diet."

How Our Bodies Undermine Exercise

Several years ago, a researcher named Herman Pontzer was studying the Hadza, a traditional hunter-gatherer tribe in northern Tanzania. The Hadza walk long distances each day and do a lot of hard, physical labor just to survive. Yet when Pontzer conducted metabolic tests on the tribesmen, he was stunned: They burned no more calories on an average day than did sedentary people back in the USA.

Pontzer continued his research when he returned to the States, and he has figured out why so many joggers, cyclists, and triathletes are still overweight: When he and his team looked at exercisers who had moderate activity levels, they found that those people burned about 200 calories more per day than people who were completely sedentary. But when they looked at exercisers with higher levels of activity, they found no increase in energy expenditure. "The most physically active people expended the same amount of calories each day as people who were only moderately active," Pontzer reported. Indeed, he suspects that once people exceed 200 calories per day in exercise, the body begins to adapt, resetting its resting metabolism to a lower point to stop weight loss. So while working out will grant you some initial impact, in short order, your body will pump the brakes on weight loss and begin hoarding extra fat the way a congressman hoards his corporate donors' private cell numbers.

If you burn off more than 200 calories a day through exercise, your metabolism will begin to slow to conserve calories and stop weight loss.

This is part of our hardwiring for survival. And there's plenty of other proof that exercise can backfire for weight loss. In a 2009 UK study, researchers put 58 sedentary, overweight, and/or obese people on a 12-week aerobic exercise program in which they worked out five times a week at 70 percent of their maximum heart rate for as long as it took to burn 500 calories per session. That's 2,500 calories a week, or enough to burn off more than 8.5 pounds during the 12-week study.

At least, it should have been. But while all of the participants showed significant increases in aerobic conditioning, lower blood pressure, and improved mood, nearly half of the participants lost little if any weight. So while aerobic exercise is great for your overall health, it's not the path to fat loss. The reason: a tricky bodily process known as "adaptive thermogenesis." While exercise may spur a quick burst of weight loss, your body soon resets its metabolism to compensate, ensuring that all of your efforts don't whittle away the body mass it worked so hard to build up. In fact, one study in the *American Journal of Clinical Nutrition* found that after weight loss, the reductions in calorie burn "persist over an extended period of time—perhaps indefinitely."

Part of that decrease in calorie burn comes from a loss of muscle mass, since the body prefers burning off muscle when it's under stress (as it is when you're exercising and restricting calories) and holding onto fat; that way, it's prepared in case the famine it's sensing gets worse. (Sadly, we're evolved to survive, not to look good in a swimsuit.)

But another reason weight loss falls off is that, when you restrict calories, as most diets require you to do, you trigger a decline in the hormone leptin, the "I'm full" hormone. Your body secretes leptin to tell your brain that your energy tank is topped off and there's no reason to raise your hand for seconds. But when leptin levels decline, you become hungrier and your body lowers the output of your thyroid gland and decreases the adrenalin your body naturally produces—all of which serves to keep you moving more slowly and preserving body fat, according to a 2013 study in the *International Journal of Obesity*.

Burning calories through exercise upsets this system, as well. First, leptin is secreted by your fat cells; when they begin to shrink, they produce less of it. As a result, your brain keeps getting the message that your tank needs to be topped off, so you keep going back to the buffet table. In fact, you're actually more likely to overeat when you lose weight because your brain becomes less sensitive to leptin signaling. And several studies have shown that the more calories you burn through exercise, the more you tend to eat during the rest of the day to compensate.

You cannot outrun a bad diet.

A 2015 study in the journal *Obesity Reviews* found that more than one-third of the weight we lose through traditional weight-loss plans will return within a year, and almost all of it will be back within three to five years, in part because of the disruption in leptin signaling. The Belly Melt Diet prevents that sort of rebound by increasing the amount of protein you eat—a step that maintains leptin levels and keeps you from growing hungry.

That's why the 7-Day Belly Melt Diet won't have you sweating off the pounds or skipping meals. Instead, you'll use the weight-loss power of protein, fat, flavonoids, and the metabolism-boosting benefits of interval training and strength training to strip away pounds and keep them off—all while burning no more than 200 calories a day extra (the maximum you can burn without triggering your body's "hold onto that fat!" mechanism).

You'll learn how to do the One Minute Morning Energizer and some easy resistance training exercises in Chapter 11. But first, let's explore what happens to your body when you eat more protein.

The Power of Protein

Learn the ways this marvelous macronutrient stifles hunger and burns fat.

SOME RESEARCHERS ARE CALLING it the "Holy Grail of weight loss," a solution that allows people to lose fat while retaining—and even growing—metabolism-boosting muscle tissue. And the way to make it happen has become clearer than ever: Eat more protein.

As you read in the previous chapter, one of the reasons rapid weight loss is often frowned upon is that when we set out to shed pounds quickly, our bodies would prefer to burn muscle rather than fat. It's a defense mechanism we developed over centuries of living through drought, famine, shipwrecks, plagues, and opposing warlords laying siege to our castles. The very thing that makes muscle so good at keeping our metabolisms revving—its ability to eat up calories—is what makes our bodies jettison it when we diet and exercise.

See, muscle burns more calories than fat does, about three times as much. And that's not just when you're moving, but even when you're sitting still. Unlike, say, sprinting through the airport, which requires an instant burst of energy, just resting your bones draws down on your fat banks slowly and steadily, like a hidden service fee, constantly tapping your fat stores and keeping them in check.

Plus, muscles do something else that helps reduce fat: Muscles store energy. When you lift a bag of groceries, go for a bike ride, or flee a charging rhino, your muscles quickly burn up energy that they've stored (in the form of glycogen). After you're done lifting, biking, or fleeing, your fat-storage hormones are subdued because your body wants to use any incoming calories to replenish those stores of glycogen in your muscle that exercise has depleted. So building muscle, and working that muscle, robs your fat stores of the ability to grow larger.

When people panic and decide they want to lose fat fast, they go on crash diets, restricting calories and doubling down on aerobics classes. Unfortunately, the one thing that crash dieting does very effectively is erode muscle.

Protein to the Rescue

How, then, can we enjoy the benefits of rapid weight loss without setting ourselves up for muscle loss and longterm weight gain? The answer is protein.

Protein helps you burn fat in three ways. First, it's the building block of muscle, and you already know that muscle burns fat. Feeding your muscles helps them grow and fight back against the forces of fleshiness. Second, the very act of eating protein actually burns calories. As much as 20 to 35 percent of the calories you eat in the form of protein are burned up just digesting the protein itself. Carbs and fat burn up no more than 5 to 15 percent of their calories. And third, protein keeps you fuller longer—in part because that intense digestive process means your body perceives you as being satiated. In a 2013 study published in the journal *Appetite,* women were fed low, moderate, or high-protein afternoon snacks. Those who ate the snack with the most protein had the lowest levels of hunger, and they waited longer to eat again than those who ate lower-protein snacks did.

So the goal, then, is to use protein to increase calorie burn and protect muscle while also tapping the power of flavonoids to strip away fat. And now we know exactly how to do it, thanks to a breakthrough 2016 study in the *American Journal of Clinical Nutrition.* Researchers at McMasters University in Toronto, Canada, put two sets of obese young men on intense weight-loss programs. Half of the subjects ate diets that were 15 percent protein, while the other half ate 35 percent of their calories from protein. Then both groups underwent intense fitness regimens, working out six days a week. After four weeks, both groups lost weight, but the men in the high-protein-diet group actually gained muscle while losing 11 to 12 pounds of fat. The men on the lower-protein diets lost about the same amount of weight, but their weight loss came from muscle as well as fat, setting them up for rebound weight gain in the future.

In other words, doubling down on protein as you strive to lose weight rapidly means you'll preserve your metabolism. You'll also protect yourself against the potential ravages of rebound weight gain. That's why the Belly Melt Diet puts a premium on meat, fish, eggs, dairy, and other sources high in this essential muscle builder.

Fire Up Your Fat Furnace

Protecting your muscle—ensuring that you'll keep your rapid weight-loss benefits for years to come—is just one of the many ways in which protein helps keep you slim, fit, and healthy. For example:

- **Protein puts your fat-burning metabolism into overdrive.** It steals energy away from fat cells—specifically belly fat cells—in order to sustain itself. And digesting protein burns up calories. Further evidence of that: A 2012 study in the *International Journal of Obesity* found that obese adults who ate three servings of yogurt each day as part of a reduced-calorie diet lost 22 percent more weight and 61 percent more body fat compared to those who didn't have the yogurt.

- **You'll feel less hungry, and have fewer food cravings.** Protein keeps you fuller longer—in part because that intense digestive process means your body perceives you as being satiated. A study published in the *American Journal of Clinical Nutrition* found that a high-protein meal increases satiety by suppressing the hunger-stimulating hormone ghrelin. That doesn't happen with a meal high in carbs. And a 2014 review of studies in the journal *ARYA Artherosclerosis* found that while restrictive diets in general tend to cause a decline in leptin, if those diets have high enough levels of protein, leptin activity can actually increase—meaning you'll feel less hunger even as you consume fewer calories.

- **You'll keep losing weight—even after you stop the 7-Day Belly Melt Diet.** Following this high-protein plan for just a short time may set you up for months of continued weight loss! In a study in the *International Journal of Obesity*, researchers found that dieters who ate a low-calorie, high-protein diet for eight weeks lost an average of 24 pounds. But unlike those in the trial who ate a low--protein, low-calorie diet, those in the high-protein group continued to lose weight—an average of 5 percent more—after the study was over. And after six months, members of the high-protein group had kept off all of their weight.

An Egg-Ceptional Protein

One of the richest sources of clean protein, eggs are also an easy, cheap, and versatile way to boost your daily protein profile. Scrambled, poached, over easy, or even over a burger, eggs are powerfully nutritious, containing the highest biological value of the muscle-building, hunger-busting macronutrient, thanks to their having all nine essential amino acids and four non-essential aminos. Low in calories (70 to 85 per) and high in protein (6 g per), the humble egg has come into its own as one of the key foods for helping people lose pounds. Studies have shown that people who replace high-carb breakfasts with egg-based meals tend to lose weight without feeling deprived. That's because protein digests more slowly and keeps blood sugar from spiking and causing cravings. Eggs are loaded with amino acids, antioxidants, and healthy fats. Don't just reach for the whites, though; the yolks boast a fat-fighting nutrient called choline, so opting for whole eggs can be even more helpful. Here's a summary of 12 beneficial effects of adding the incredible edible egg to your diet:

- **You'll boost your immune system.** If you don't want to play chicken with infections, viruses, and diseases, add an egg or two to your diet daily. Just one large egg contains almost a quarter (22 percent) of your RDA of selenium, a nutrient that helps support your immune system and regulate thyroid hormones. Kids especially should eat eggs. If children and adolescents don't get enough selenium, they could develop Keshan disease and Kashin-Beck disease, two conditions that can affect the heart, bones, and joints.

- **You'll improve your cholesterol profile.** There are three ideas about cholesterol that practically everyone knows: 1) High cholesterol is a bad thing; 2) There are "good" and "bad" kinds of cholesterol; 3) Eggs contain plenty of the stuff. Doctors are generally most concerned with the ratio of good cholesterol (HDL) to bad cholesterol (LDL) in the blood. One large egg contains 212 mg of cholesterol, but this doesn't mean that eating eggs raises the level of the bad kind in the blood. The body constantly produces cholesterol on its own, and a large body of evidence indicates that eggs can actually improve your cholesterol profile. How? They seem to raise HDL cholesterol while increasing the size of LDL particles (which may make them less dangerous).

- **You'll reduce your risk of heart disease.** Not only have eggs been found to not increase risk of coronary heart disease, but they might actually decrease your risk. LDL cholesterol became known as bad cholesterol because LDL particles transport their fat molecules into artery walls, and drive atherosclerosis, basically the gumming up of the arteries. (HDL particles, by contrast, can remove fat molecules from artery walls.) But not all LDL particles are made equal, and there are various subtypes that differ in size. Bigger is definitely better—many studies have shown that people who have predominantly small, dense LDL particles have a higher risk of heart disease than people who have mostly larger LDL particles. Here's the best part: Even if eggs tend to raise LDL cholesterol in some people, studies show that they help LDL particles change from small and dense to large, slashing the risk of cardiovascular problems.

- **You'll have more get-up-and-go.** Just one egg contains about 15 percent of your RDA of vitamin B2, also called riboflavin. It's just one of the eight B vitamins that help the body convert food into fuel, which in turn is used to produce energy.

- **Your skin and hair will improve.** In addition to vitamin B2, eggs are rich in skin-loving B5 (pantothenic acid) and nerve- and blood-feeding B12 (cobalamin). The yolks contain B7 (biotin), which promotes hair and scalp health.

- **You'll protect your brain.** Eggs are brain food. That's largely because of an essential nutrient called choline. It's a component of cell membranes and is required to synthesize acetylcholine, a neurotransmitter. Studies show that a lack of choline has been linked to neurological disorders and decreased cognitive function. Shockingly, more than 90 percent of Americans eat less than the daily recommended amount of choline, found a U.S. dietary survey.

- **You'll save your life.** Among the lesser-known amazing things the body can do: It can make 11 essential amino acids that are necessary to sustain life. Thing is, there are 20 amino acids total that your body needs. Guess where the other nine can be found? That's right. A lack of those nine amino acids can lead to muscle wasting, decreased immune response, weakness, fatigue, and changes to the texture of your skin and hair.

- **You'll have less stress and anxiety.** Being deficient in the nine amino acids that can be found in an egg can have mental effects. A 2004 study in *Proceedings of the National Academy of Sciences* described how supplementing a population's diet with lysine significantly reduced anxiety and stress levels, possibly by modulating mood-regulating serotonin in the nervous system.

- **You'll protect your peepers.** Two antioxidants found in eggs—lutein and zeaxanthin—have powerful protective effects on the eyes. You won't find them in a carton of Egg Beaters—they only exist in the yolk. Both significantly reduce the risk of macular degeneration and cataracts, which are among the leading causes of vision impairment and blindness in the elderly. In a study published in the *American Journal of Clinical Nutrition*, participants who ate 1.3 egg yolks per day for four-and-a-half weeks increased their blood levels of zeaxanthin by 114 to 142 percent and upped their lutein by 28 to 50 percent!

- **You'll improve your bones and teeth.** Eggs are one of the few natural sources of vitamin D, which is important for the health and strength of bones and teeth. It does its beneficial work in the body primarily by aiding the absorption of calcium. (Calcium, incidentally, is important for a healthy heart, a high-functioning colon, and a strong metabolism.)

- **You'll feel fuller and eat less.** Eggs are such a good source of quality protein that all other sources of protein are measured against them. (Eggs get a perfect score of 100.) Many studies have demonstrated the effect of high-protein foods on appetite. Simply put, they take the edge off. You might not be surprised to learn that eggs score high on a scale called the Satiety Index, a measure of how much foods contribute to the feeling of fullness.

- **You'll lose fat.** Largely because of their high Satiety Index score, eggs have been linked with fat loss. A study of their ability to sate produced some remarkable results: Over an eight-week period, people ate a breakfast of either two eggs or a bagel, which contained the same amount of calories. The egg group lost 65 percent more body weight and 16 percent more body fat, experienced a 61 percent greater reduction in BMI, and saw a 34 percent greater reduction in waist circumference! While you'll be starting your day with a smoothie, consider fitting satiating eggs into other parts of your day.

- **You'll protect your liver.** B vitamins aren't the only ovular micronutrients that contribute to eggs' beneficial effects on liver health. Eggs are also rich in the nutrient choline. (One large egg contains between 117 and 147 milligrams of the nutrient, depending on your cooking method of choice). A recent scientific review explained that choline deficiency is linked to the accumulation of hepatic lipid, which can cause nonalcoholic fatty liver disease. Luckily, a *Journal of Nutrition* study found that a higher dietary choline intake may be associated with a lower risk of the disease in women.

- **You'll lower your risk of type 2 diabetes.** Another side effect of choline deficiency and the subsequent accumulation of hepatic lipid is an increase in your risk of insulin resistance and type 2 diabetes, so getting enough of the nutrient brings down your risk.

- **You'll reduce inflammation.** Eggs are a major source of dietary phospholipids, bioactive compounds that, studies show, have widespread effects on inflammation. A recent review published in the journal *Nutrients* connected dietary intake of egg phospholipids and choline with a reduction in countless biomarkers of inflammation. Lowering inflammation has widespread health benefits that range from lowering risk of cardiovascular disease to improving the body's ability to break down fat.

Surprising Sources of Protein

Man cannot live on eggs alone. Nor can woman. And we all may want to limit our consumption of meats. Fortunately, you can also find the supernutrient hiding in some unexpected places. These surprising sources of protein can open up an expansive array of meal opportunities.

Avocados 4 grams protein per fruit

High in healthy monounsaturated fats, avocados also deliver a surprising dose of protein. Another reason to make guacamole your go-to appetizer.

Broccoli rabe 3.3 grams protein per ⅓ cup

This bitter cousin to your bland, boring broccoli has one of the highest protein-per-calorie ratios in the plant world: 1 gram of protein for every 8.7 calories. A serving will give you 3.3 grams for just 28 calories—that's more protein than a spoonful of peanut butter.

Chickpea pasta 14 grams protein per 2 ounces

While white pasta, like other low-protein, low-fiber grains, is off your plate for the next 7 days, chickpea pasta is an incredible cheat that lets you enjoy the protein and fiber of chickpeas and the satisfying carb feel of noodles. Banza pasta, made with chickpeas, has twice as much protein as regular pasta, while also providing 8 grams of fiber and only about half the carbs of your average pasta dinner. And it's gluten-free!

Cocoa powder (unsweetened)
2 grams protein per 2 tablespoons

Mix some cocoa powder into your smoothie for a boost of more than just decadent chocolatey taste. In addition to delivering a gram of protein for every 12 calories, it will also give you 4 grams of fat-burning fiber and 20 percent of your daily value for the essential muscle mineral manganese.

Falafel 2.5 grams protein per falafel

They look like crab cakes that have escaped from a cocktail party, but falafels are little balls of chickpeas and herbs that deliver a gram of protein for every 25 calories.

Flaxmeal 2 grams protein per 2 tablespoons

You may think of flax for its fiber content and rich omega-3 fatty acid profile, but flax is a potent protein source, as well. Two tablespoons of the meal gives you 2 grams of musclebuilding protein as well as 4 grams of metabolism-enhancing fiber. Blend some into your morning F.L.A.V.O.R. smoothie!

Grapefruit 2 grams protein per fruit

Plenty of studies have shown that grapefruit stands alone as a particularly powerful weight-loss food. One study in the *Journal of Medical Food* found that people who ate half a fresh grapefruit a day lost 3½ pounds in 12 weeks despite making no changes in diet or exercise. Its metabolism-boosting flavonoids are only further enhanced by the fruit's protein levels.

Green beans 6 grams protein per ½ cup

They may be French, but green beans aren't rich in the Julia Child French cooking kind of way; they'll keep you lean with a solid gram of vegetable protein for every 18 calories.

Hubbard squash 2.5 grams protein per ½ cup

The big, blue, gnarly looking squash that shows up every autumn harbors a secret stash of metabolism-boosting protein. The seeds deliver 8 grams of protein per ¼ cup once you've roasted and salted them, but the squash meat itself will supply another few grams. Spice it up with cinnamon and serve it as an alternative to sweet potatoes.

Hummus 6 grams protein per ½ cup

Perhaps the very best thing you can dip a chip into, hummus delivers a gram of protein for each 36 calories. Made from chickpeas and olive oil, it's as healthy as a food can get.

Mushrooms 4 grams protein per 1 cup

You may know about the protein-packing power of portobello mushrooms because they show up in place of burgers at some restaurants. But most mushrooms deliver about 4 grams of protein per serving, for less than 40 calories. They're also a great source of selenium, a mineral that's essential for proper muscle function.

Passion Fruit 2.5 grams protein per ½ cup

Passion fruit delivers a surprising dose of protein thanks to its edible seeds; a half cup also gives you 12 grams of fiber and more than half a day's vitamin C.

Peanuts 9 grams protein per ¼ cup

The king nut (though it's technically a legume) when it comes to protein is the humble peanut. In fact, it tops tree nuts like pecans (2.5 grams), cashews (5 grams), and even almonds (8 grams) in the protein power rankings. Peanuts are also a terrific source of mood-boosting folate.

Pistachios 6.5 grams protein per ¼ cup

All nuts are high in protein, but pistachios may have additional metabolic powers, making them one of the best-ever high-protein snacks. A recent study by scientists in India looked at 60 middle-aged men who were at risk for diabetes and heart disease. They divided them into two groups and had them eat similar diets, except that one of the groups got 20 percent of their daily calories from pistachios. The group that ate the pistachios had smaller waists at the end of the study; their cholesterol score dropped by 15 points, and their blood sugar numbers improved, as well.

Pomegranate 5 grams protein per fruit

You might not think of fruit when you think of protein, but pomegranates stand out as protein powerhouses. The reason: The protein is stored in the seeds of the fruit. Don't make the mistake of thinking that Pom Wonderful will give you the same benefits, however—it's full of sugars.

Pumpkin seeds 9 grams protein per ounce

A good source of protein, healthy fats, and fiber, these squash seeds keep you feeling full and energized longer, and contain manganese, magnesium, phosphorus, and zinc, which support muscle growth. Toss them into salads.

Spinach 5 grams protein per 1 cup, cooked

One cup of the leafy superfood has nearly as much protein as a hard-boiled egg—for half the calories. Looking to get the biggest nutritional bang for your buck? Be sure to steam your spinach instead of eating it raw. Steaming helps retain the green's vitamins and makes it easier for the body to absorb the its calcium content.

Spirulina 8 grams protein per tablespoon

Spirulina is a blue-green algae that's typically dried and sold in powdered form, although you can also buy spirulina flakes and tablets. Dried spirulina is about 60 percent protein and, unlike most plants, it's a complete protein, meaning it can be converted directly into muscle in the body. A tablespoon delivers 8 grams of metabolism-boosting protein for just 43 calories, plus half a day's allotment of vitamin B12.

Sweet peas 3 grams protein per ½ cup

Like all legumes, peas are great sources of protein. But you get an additional boost from sweet peas, the kind that come in their own edible pods (also known as *mange tout*). Eat them raw or steam them and top with a dab of butter and some sea salt. You'll get a gram of protein for every 15 calories you consume.

Tempeh 16 grams protein per ½ cup

Mas macho than its softer cousin, tofu, tempeh is made from soybeans, rather than soy milk. As a result, it's closer to a whole food, and keeps more of its protein, about 50 percent more than tofu.

Vegan protein powder 15 to 20 grams protein per scoop

More and more, research is showing that when we add plant proteins to our diets, our bodies respond by shedding fat. In a 2015 study in the *Journal of Diabetes Investigation,* researchers discovered that patients who ingested higher amounts of vegetable protein were far less susceptible to metabolic syndrome (a disease that ought to be renamed "diabolic syndrome"—it's basically a combination of high cholesterol, high blood sugar, and obesity). That means eating whole foods from vegetables—and supplementing with vegan protein powder—is one of the best ways to keep extra weight at bay. A second study in *Nutrition Journal* found that "plant protein intakes may play a role in preventing obesity." Vega One All-in-One Nutritional Shake, Vega Sport Performance Protein, and Sunwarrior Warrior Blend are three we love.

Wheatgrass powder 2 grams protein per 1.25 tablespoons

What doesn't wheatgrass offer for a mere 30 calories? Even a tiny dose like this packs fiber, protein, tons of vitamin A and K, folic acid, manganese, iodine, and chlorophyll, to name a few. You don't need to know what each nutrient does for you; just know that a single tablespoon will have you operating at peak performance levels.

Shut-off Switches
Eat these 7 foods that silence hunger hormones fast.

There's a crybaby in your gut. It's called ghrelin, remember, the "I'm hungry" hormone? When your stomach is empty—or thinks it is—it secretes ghrelin, which causes hunger by sending signals to the brain, urging you to launch a search-and-destroy mission aimed at any nearby bags of Doritos.

Your belly's babysitter? Leptin, an appetite suppressor that signals to your brain when you're full and tells it to stop eating. But just as we can develop an insensitivity to another food-related hormone, insulin, so too can we develop a resistance to leptin, researchers say. The result: Your hunger doesn't shut off naturally, and you continue to eat even when you're full.

The same dietary factors that lead to insulin resistance—high-sugar, high-calorie foods lacking in protein and fiber—can cause our brain's appetite-suppression mechanisms to go awry. But fortunately, some foods have the opposite effect, improving our hunger management not just in the short term, but over the long haul, as well. To whittle your middle down rapidly, eat more of these foods that turn off the appetite tap fast, and keep it off for hours.

1. Apples
As you know, apples are an excellent source of hunger-busting fiber, so don't feel constrained by the whole "one-a-day" thing. A recent study at Wake Forest Baptist Medical Center found that for every additional 10 grams of soluble fiber eaten per day, a study subject's belly fat was reduced by 3.7 percent over five years. And research at the University of Western Australia found that levels of antioxidant flavonoids in the Pink Lady variety ranked among the highest of any apple, making them tops in fighting inflammation and protecting heart health. Other stars: Red Delicious, Northern Spy, Cortland, Mutsu, Macintosh.

2. Apple cider vinegar
White vinegar's sassier cousin is composed mostly of acetic acid, which has been shown to delay gastric emptying and slow the release of sugar into the bloodstream, according to a study published in the journal *BMC*

Gastroenterology. One study among pre-diabetics found the addition of 2 tablespoons of apple cider vinegar to a high-carb meal reduced the subsequent rise in blood sugar by 34 percent!

3. Artichokes

Ghrelin is suppressed when your stomach is full, so eating satiating high-fiber foods is a nobrainer. Leafy greens are an excellent choice, but don't overlook the humble artichoke, which contains almost twice as much fiber as kale (10.3 g per medium artichoke, or 40 percent of the daily fiber the average woman needs). Artichokes are also one of the foods highest in the prebiotic inulin, which feeds your good gut bacteria, a.k.a. probiotics. (When your gut health goes awry, so do your leptin and ghrelin levels.) Other foods high in inulin are garlic, onions, leeks, and bananas.

4. Eggs

Breakfast is no longer considered a nutritional make-or-break, but waking up to a protein-rich meal can set your fat-burning pace for your entire day. In a study of 21 men published in the journal *Nutrition Research*, half were fed a breakfast of bagels while half ate eggs. The egg group was observed to have a lower response to ghrelin, was less hungry three hours later, and consumed fewer calories for the next 24 hours!

Bonus: Egg yolks contain choline, a nutrient with powerful fat-burning properties. While the Belly Melt Diet calls for smoothies each morning, consider fitting eggs into other parts of your day.

5. Halibut

Fish has a ton of benefits—it's high in omega-3 acids, which reduce inflammation throughout the body and allow leptin to communicate efficiently with the brain—and halibut is especially great. The Satiety Index of Common Foods ranks halibut the second most filling food (bested only by boiled potatoes). The study's authors attribute that to halibut's high protein content and levels of tryptophan; the latter produces serotonin, one of the hormones that curbs hunger. Halibut is also one of the best sources for methionine, a nutrient that reverses the gene signals for insulin resistance and obesity.

6. Oysters

Resolve to do more prying. Oysters are one of the best food sources of zinc, a mineral that works with leptin to regulate appetite. Research shows that overweight people tend to have higher levels of leptin and lower levels of zinc than slimmer folk. A study published in the journal *Life Sciences* found that taking zinc supplements could increase leptin production in obese men by 142 percent! A half dozen oysters only has 43 calories but provides 21 percent of your RDA of iron—deficiencies of which have been linked to a significant increase in fat gene expression.

7. Rooibos tea

Made from the leaves of the "red bush" plant, rooibos tea is grown exclusively in the small Cederberg region of South Africa. What makes it a winner at the Hunger Games? A flavonoid called aspalathin. According to research, the compound can reduce stress hormones that trigger hunger and prompt fat storage and are linked to hypertension, metabolic syndrome, cardiovascular disease, insulin resistance, and type 2 diabetes.

The Belly Bulgers

Avoid these calorie-dense foods that cause weight gain.

WHEN YOU FILL your plate with F.L.A.V.O.R. foods, you take cravings and bingeing out of the equation. Belly-filling, fiber-rich vegetables and fruits and satisfying proteins replace fast-burning carbohydrates that spike blood sugar and trigger more intense cravings and rapid-fire munching

That's the key to rapid weight loss: Replace the calorie-dense stuff that encourages you to eat more calorie-dense stuff. Simple. Or it should be. What makes rapid weight loss not so simple is having lots of high-calorie, high-carb, mostly processed packaged foods and snacks lying around your kitchen whispering sweet "eat me's" in your ears. Those foods are often heavy on trans fats, added sugars, and added sodium—three things that do a number on your health and make it difficult to lose weight. So, get rid of them. Banish those temptations. You can't mindlessly eat a whole bag of potato chips or a pint of salted-caramel-laced vanilla ice cream if those snacks aren't in your home.

One of the best things you can do to speed up weight loss is to grab a heavy-duty plastic trash bag and do a clean sweep of your pantry and refrigerator, tossing out the snacks, sodas, juices, baked goods, and other highly processed, high-calorie munchies. At the very least, keep that stuff off the kitchen counter, out of eyesight and arm's reach.

In a 2015 study called "Slim by Design: Kitchen Counter Correlates of Obesity" in the journal *Health Education and Behavior*, researchers from Cornell University, Ohio State University, and VTT Technical Research Centre of Finland found a clear relationship between a person's body mass index (or BMI, a measure of body fat) and the foods found on his or her kitchen counter. Analyzing more than 700 households, the researchers found that the presence of processed foods like candy, cereal, soft drinks, and dried fruit on a home's kitchen counters correlated with higher body weight in the people living in the home, while fresh fruit on a home's kitchen counters correlated with lower BMI in the occupants of the home. "It's your basic 'see-food diet'—you eat what you see," says lead researcher Brian Wansink, professor and director of the Cornell University Food & Brand Lab.

Analysis of a subset of that study showed that women who had breakfast cereal on their counter weighed on average 20 pounds more than women who did not have cereal in plain sight. Those who had soft drinks sitting out weighed 24 to 26 pounds more, while women who had fruit sitting a bowl on their counter weighed an average of 13 pounds less.

20 Temptation Foods to Dump

1. Breakfast Cereals and Even Certain Instant Oatmeals

Generally, breakfast cereals are boxes of empty sugar calories. Sure, there are some that are high in dietary fiber, but even these can be loaded with sugar. Steel-cut oats are generally good as a snack or breakfast option for the maintenance phase of the program in this book, but even the hallowed oatmeal can be compromised with secret additions. You need to be wary of the ingredients list. As you go through your packaged foods (including instant oatmeals—beware of Quaker Instant Oatmeal Fruit & Cream, for example) keep an eye peeled for trans fats, corn syrup, and added sugars. "Often listed as hydrogenated or partially hydrogenated oils, synthetically engineered trans fats increase your bad (LDL) cholesterol levels and decrease your good (HDL) cholesterol levels, upping your risk of heart attack and stroke," says Eugenia Gianos, MD, cardiologist, who is the co-clinical director at the Center for the Prevention of Cardiovascular Disease at NYU Langone Medical Center.

QUICK TIP: If your oats need a flavor boost, add fresh fruits, a touch of honey, or an ounce of nuts to your bowl instead.

2. Canned Cream-Based Soups

Most canned soups are loaded with sodium, but the cream-based ones carry other things among their empty calories—fillers like hydrolyzed proteins, food dyes, and corn syrup. Also, the cans the soups are stored in are too often laced with bisphenol A (BPA), an industrial chemical used in various food and beverage containers. BPA is thought to pose some health risks in fetuses' and young children's brain development.

QUICK TIP: Look for protein-based soups like black bean soup, which is high in fiber. Avoid canned soups. Add avocado to get some healthy fat. And look for reduced-sodium versions.

3. Canned Vegetables

Americans typically eat only one-third of the recommended daily intakes, so you may be surprised to hear us knock any form of vegetable. Unfortunately, we've got to go there. Why? BPA in the lining of the can.

QUICK TIP: Try going with fresh or frozen veggies, which tend to be healthier and free of salt and preservatives, too.

4. Deli Meats

The connection between salt-, sugar-, and chemical-laden processed meats and chronic disease risk is strong and consistent in scientific research. If you eat meat, it should be pure—just as you want your own muscles to be, advises David L. Katz, MD, MPH, who is director of the Yale University Prevention Research Center and president of the American College of Lifestyle Medicine.

5. Egg Beaters

"This is as far removed from a natural egg as you can get," says Dana James CDN, a nutritionist from Food Coach NYC. "Heat-pasteurized and made from factory-farmed eggs, this product is processed so much that makers actually have to add in synthetic vitamins to boost its nutrient density.

QUICK TIP: "Go for the real thing instead," says James. Choline, a nutrient found in eggs, lean meats, seafood, and collard greens, attacks the gene mechanism that triggers your body to store fat around your liver.

6. Frozen French Fries

There's something almost magical about the effects of fried spuds on your body's fat-storage system. One long-term Harvard University study found that people who ate fries regularly gained more than three pounds of body weight every four years; over the course of the study, the French fry eaters gained 15 pounds of belly flab from fries alone!

7. Fruit Juice

"Talk about turning a good food bad," says Leah Kaufman, MS, RD, CDN, a New York City–based registered dietitian. "When you transform produce into juice, you take away its fiber—one of the major benefits of consuming whole fruits and vegetables. What you wind up with is a drink that's so concentrated with sweetness, it can have as much sugar as a soda."

QUICK TIP: Eat your fruit whole to get the fiber and more vitamins than juice has. More and more research has begun to show that some fruits are actually better at fighting belly fat than others. Which ones? Look for red or reddish: Raspberries, strawberries, blueberries—they're packed with polyphenols, powerful natural chemicals that can actually stop fat from forming.

8. Granola

"This is one of our leading health-food impostors!" says Lisa Moskovitz, RD, founder of The NY Nutrition Group. "One tiny cup of granola has nearly 600 calories, 30 grams of fat, and 24 grams of sugar. That's the equivalent of starting your morning with two slices of cheesecake."

9. High-Calorie Bottled Fruit Smoothies

A fruit smoothie sounds like a virtuous choice for an afternoon pick-me-up, but be forewarned: Many store-bought options are blended with high-calorie dairy bases and cheap sweeteners that make them more dessert-like than diet friendly. Some contain as many as 440 calories, nearly a third of what the average woman on a 1,500-calorie weight-loss diet needs in an entire day. Not to mention 96 grams of sugar—that's more than you'll find in seven scoops of sherbet.

10. Ketchup

A measly two tablespoons has up to eight grams of sugar and 40 calories. And most of those calories come from high-fructose corn syrup, which has been shown to increase appetite and, over time, lead to obesity and diabetes.

11. Low-Fat Packaged Baked Goods

Typically, these items are extensively processed and are packed with chemicals that are added to try to achieve the consistency or reproduce the flavor of the full-fat models. You are better off indulging in a smaller portion of a food naturally high in fat or sugar than ingesting an artificial substitute. And in most cases, the real deal tastes better, is more satisfying, and doesn't cause the gastrointestinal upset that can be associated with highly processed foods.

12. Nutella

It may sound nuts, but this "hazelnut spread" is primarily made of sugar and palm oil with almost no actual nuts. So don't be fooled into thinking it's worth space in your pantry. With more than 20 grams of added sugar and only two grams of protein, the spread just winds up at your waist.

13. Nutrient-Stripped Bread

If you have white bread in your cupboard, feed it to the ducks at the lake. Then, go to a health-food store and score some sprouted grain bread. It's heartier, tastes better, and is loaded with fiber. You need more fiber. We all do. White bread, by contrast, has been bleached and stripped of its bran and germ, the elements of the grain that contain beneficial nutrients. "White bread isn't very filling, has almost no nutritional value, and is converted into sugar once you eat it," says Jim White RD, ACSM, owner of Jim White Fitness and Nutrition Studios. "Like table sugar, it then spikes insulin levels, which promotes fat storage,"

Stop Drinking Yourself Fat

The easiest way to cut calories is to stop drinking sugar.

The third-largest source of food calories in the typical American diet isn't food at all: It's soft drinks. In fact, Americans get more calories from soft drinks every day than from meat, dairy, or anything other than baked goods. In fact, one in four of us gets more than 200 calories a day from beverages, and one in every 20 gets more than 560 calories a day! Simply cutting those calories out could save you between 21 and 58 pounds of fat a year.

Soft drinks don't just mess with our waistlines by adding lots of empty calories. The real damage lies in the way that they undermine our belly biome—creating the worst possible environment for our good gut bacteria while also providing comfort to the enemy: sugar. The sweet stuff is the preferred food of the unhealthy gut bugs that wreak havoc on our systems, causing inflammation, bloating, and weight gain. Address your drinking problem and you'll make bold strides toward a lean, flat belly, a healthy gut, and a better life. In fact, if you drink just one or two sodas, sweetened iced teas, or flavored waters a day, consider how much you have to gain by switching to sparkling or plain water or homebrewed green tea:

- **You'll stop waistline creep.** We don't get fat all of a sudden. We get fat slowly. In a two-decade-long study of 200,000 people, the people who increased their intake of sugary beverages by just one a day were five pounds heavier than those who abstained.

- **You'll protect your kids.** For each 12-ounce sweetened beverage a child consumes per day, his or her risk of becoming obese over the next 18 months increases by 60 percent, according to a study in the *Lancet*.

- **You'll slash your risk of diabetes.** People who consume just one or two sugary drinks a day have a 26 percent greater risk of diabetes than those who don't indulge in them, according to a study in the journal *Diabetes Care*.

- **You'll avoid that date with a heart attack.** A study that followed 40,000 men for 20 years found that those who drank just one can of a sugary beverage a day had a 20 percent higher risk of dying from heart attack than those who drank none.

  Drinks to avoid include sugar-added sodas, iced teas, and energy drinks; flavored coffee drinks; and fruit and vegetable juices as well as juice cocktails.

  Adult drinks to avoid: all of them—wine, beer, cocktails. If your goal is to lose your belly as rapidly as possible, there can be no room for alcohol, a big source of empty calories that actually encourages fat storage. This doesn't mean you can't have a glass of wine ever again. Just wait until you've realized your goal weight and shape and embarked on your maintenance phase. Otherwise, your best chance of meeting your bikini deadline is to avoid alcohol.

CONTINUED FROM PAGE 75

says White. Don't get caught up in phrases like, "made with whole grains." This catchy phrase can make you think your bread is a healthy choice, but it only means that the bread is made up of a mixture of whole-wheat flour and some other less-nutritious flour that won't benefit your health. Also, keep an eye out for the words "bleached flour" on ingredients lists, too. Bleaching adds chemicals to the bread and strips away vital nutrients.

14. Nutrition Bars

For the amount of calorie-dense carbohydrates and fat they contain, you might as well eat a candy bar. Many of these energy bars are packed with simple sugars, and they aren't quite filling enough to substitute for a meal or snack.

15. Rice Cakes

Rice cakes are an old-school diet staple. But the simple carbohydrates rank notoriously high on the glycemic index (GI)—a measure of how quickly blood rises in response to food calculated on a scale of one to 100 (rice cakes come in at 82). High-GI foods provide a rush of energy, but can leave you hungry within a few hours. Researchers at the New Balance Foundation Obesity Prevention Center found that high-GI snacks caused excessive hunger and increased activity in craving and reward area of the brain—the perfect storm for overeating and weight gain.

QUICK TIP: Adding healthy fats or protein to a meal lowers its glycemic load. Swap a two-cake mini-meal for one rice cake topped with a generous swipe of nut butter. The combo will keep you fuller for longer and has the added benefit of being a complete protein with all nine essential amino acids.

16. Roasted Almonds

Sure, roasted nuts are delicious. But the high-heat cooking method does nut'n for your waistline. One study in the journal *Food Biophysics* showed that raw almonds caused stomach acids to swell (in a good way) and were slower to be digested than roasted almonds, creating a greater feeling of fullness that lasted longer. Moreover, store-bought varieties are often roasted in oil and then tossed in salt and preservatives. Emerald Nuts Dry Roasted Almonds may be oil-free, but you'll find 18 other ingredients on the label, including monosodium glutamate (MSG), a controversial flavor enhancer linked to weight gain in some studies.

QUICK TIP: Go raw or go home. Brownie points if you opt for in-shell varieties. Named "The Pistachio Effect," research shows the act of shelling nuts can slow you down and give your body a chance to register fullness 86 calories sooner than it would otherwise.

17. Soda—Even Diet Soda

Most sodas contain phosphorus, which binds to calcium and increases calcium loss, which is terrible for bone health. Plus, a single can is filled with 40 grams of sugar—the equivalent of 20 sugar cubes—which makes it challenging for the body to maintain healthy glucose and insulin levels. And diet varieties are potentially worse. Diet sodas contain low doses of carcinogens, and their artificial sweeteners have potentially dangerous effects on the brain and metabolism.

QUICK TIP: "Vow to eat your calories instead of sipping them through a straw," advises Cheryl Forberg, RD, who was a nutritionist on *The Biggest Loser*. She says one of the most common behaviors of overweight contestants she has counseled is that they consumed large quantities of sugary sodas, cream-laden coffees, juices, and alcohol. "Ditch the sippable junk."

18. Soy Milk

Soy mimics the hormone estrogen and activates estrogen receptors in the body. For men, eating a lot of soy could possibly encourage the development of enlarged breasts.

QUICK TIP: There are plenty of other milk substitutes— like almond milk—that don't carry these potential side effects.

19. Sugary Drinks & Candy

Even the smallest sizes of sweetened coffee drinks like Starbuck's Frappuccinos pack an average of 300 to 400 calories, which would take you about 40 minutes to jog off on a treadmill. These sugary drinks are also full of artificial colorings and preservatives that have been linked to childhood attention-deficit disorders and allergic reactions. Instead of grabbing a Frappuccino, consider a tall plain latte made with organic shade-grown grounds and 2 percent milk and sprinkled with some cinnamon to add a kick without the calories.

Consuming fruit juice on occasion isn't terrible for you, but drinking it too often can have a negative impact on health and body composition. A cup of grape juice, for example, contains nearly the same amount of sugar as two Dunkin' Donuts Glazed Cake Donuts, and a large OJ from McDonald's has as much sugar as 25 Lifesavers Gummies. Processed juices also contain significant amounts of high-fructose corn syrup, which can cause weight gain and elevated cholesterol levels. And tossing back a handful of candy might not seem like a big deal, but it's the equivalent of chowing down on pure sugar.

20. Turkey Bacon

It contains 13 fewer calories per slice and slightly less saturated fat than pork bacon, but a lot more sodium, which is not good—especially if you have high blood pressure. Pork also delivers more protein and heart-healthy monounsaturated fatty acids than turkey bacon, making it a better choice.

Banish Added Sugars
Consider these ingredients hazardous to your health.

You probably already know how sugar screws up weight-loss goals: When we take in a dose of sugar, our blood sugar rises quickly. In high doses, sugar is toxic, as the pancreas reacts by shooting out insulin, a hormone that helps pull the sugar out of our bloodstream and turns it into energy that we can burn. But unless we're skiing down a mountain or leaping to spike a volleyball, there's often more energy on hand than we can burn off, so it quickly gets stored as fat.

Not only does that help bury your abs under layers of flab, but it also can help ultimately bury you under several feet of dirt. For the first time, scientists have linked the amount of sugar in a person's diet with the risk of dying from heart disease. In a study recently published in the *Journal of The American Medical Association*, people who ate between 17 and 21 percent of their calories from added sugar had a 38 percent higher risk of dying from heart disease, compared with people who consumed eight percent or less of their calories from added sugar.

New research suggests that for every five percent of total calories you consume from sweeteners, your risk of diabetes bumps up by 18 percent. "Bad" cholesterol and heart disease risk increase after only two weeks of eating corn-based sweeteners.

Now, some of the foods on the 7-Day Belly Melt Diet are high in sugars—including fructose, the form of sugar found naturally in fruit, and lactose, the sugars that are present in dairy. But those sugars come with their own posse of nutrients (like protein, fiber, and flavonoids) that allow our bodies to respond to them without experiencing the blood-sugar spikes and cholesterol and blood pressure rises that come from added sugars. And by added sugars, we mean all types of sweeteners that are added to foods, from natural ones like cane sugar, corn syrup, honey, agave, maltodextrin, and brown rice syrup to artificial ones like sucralose and aspartame. All have been linked to weight gain and other health concerns, including inflammation, insulin resistance, and overall metabolic dysfunction.

How to Follow the 7-Day Belly Melt Diet

Stick to these six simple rules for superfast success.

ANY PLAN THAT PROMISES rapid, dramatic, and effortless weight loss must be a) really complicated, b) really miserable, or c) really expensive (or a combination of all three). How else could one deliver such remarkable results?

Well, it's programs that are complicated, miserable, and expensive that actually create dietary failures. Knowing what to eat in any situation, enjoying the food you eat, and being able to sustain the program from both a financial and an emotional-reward perspective are the three keys to whether a diet will work for you.

In this chapter, you'll learn just how easy such a plan

can be. By following these six simple rules, you'll always be confident and in control, and never have to worry about whether you're on top of your diet. Weight loss is going to be remarkably easy (and delicious) as long as you stick to the plan.

LOSE YOUR BELLY RULE #1:
Eat Six Times a Day

Eating six times during the day, at regular intervals, seems to be one of the best ways to keep your metabolism revving, according to a study in the *American Journal of Clinical Nutrition*. Researchers found that when women ate six times a day, they ate fewer total calories that day, burned more of the calories they did consume, and had lower levels of both blood glucose and cholesterol than when they ate as few as three times or as many as nine times a day.

Starting off with breakfast is a critical part of that plan. A 2010 study at Dartmouth College found that eating breakfast can increase your resting metabolism by 10 percent. And a 2015 study at Tel Aviv University found that people who eat breakfast have more stable blood glucose levels through the rest of the day, regardless of what or how much they eat at their other meals.

SUCCESS TIP: Get in the habit of recording your meals and snacks in your Food Tracker in the appendix. To be honest, this takes effort, but the payoff can be big. In a large study of 1,700 people in a weight-loss program published in the *American Journal of Preventive Medicine*, researchers at the Kaiser Permanente Center for Health Research in Portland, Oregon, found that subjects who kept daily food journals lost twice as much as weight as those who didn't.

LOSE YOUR BELLY RULE #2:
Focus on the F.L.A.V.O.R. Foods

In a previous chapter, you met the F.L.A.V.O.R. foods and discovered how each one plays a significant and unique role in helping you burn away your belly fast, from the calorie-melting proteins to the belly-flattening oils to the various flavonoid-rich vegetables and fruits.

But focusing on these whole foods does something else: It crowds out the less-desirable foods that want to worm their way into your day. The more whole F.L.A.V.O.R. foods you eat, the less room there is for foods that won't carry their weight in helping you lose the weight. That's part of why you'll be eating six times a day—to ensure you never get hungry, never have cravings, and never have to resist the siren call of the office vending machine.

Eating more often and choosing nutrient-dense F.L.A.V.O.R. foods as mainstays of your diet both help to control appetite. But the third way that this plan helps to keep you full, satisfied, and burning fat is by packing your food choices with fiber. In one clinical trial, a fiber-dense fruit-based micronutrient and supplement bar was shown to improve metabolism in overweight/obese otherwise healthy adults in ways that are consistent with reduced risk of type 2 diabetes and cardiovascular disease. Consumption of the bar for two months also reduced chronic inflammation and initiated a reduction in weight and waist circumference.

A five-year study that appeared in the journal *Nutrition* found that the connection between eating more fruits and vegetables and a lower body weight was even greater when the produce-heavy diet was high in overall fiber. The takeaway? The more fruits and vegetables you eat, the more fiber you take in, the more weight you lose.

Start Each Day with a Smoothie

What's so special about smoothies? Well, first of all, they're delicious—so creamy and filling you'll wonder whether you're having breakfast or dessert. And they deliver a massive dose of fat-fighting flavonoids right when you need them: at the beginning of the day, before you take on the world of office birthday parties, vending machines, and pizza commercials. But there's something uniquely powerful about smoothies.

- In a 2012 study in *Current Nutrition and Food Science*, researchers put a group of obese adults on a regimen in which they replaced both breakfast and dinner with a high-protein, nutrient-rich smoothie. That was all: no exercise, no limit on what else they could eat. After 12 weeks, the subjects lost up to 18.5 pounds and reported significant improvements in "physical functioning, general health, vitality, and mental health."

- A high-protein diet featuring meal-replacement drinks is more effective than exercise at helping people lose weight and keep it off, according to a 2013 meta-analysis of 20 studies, which included more than 3,000 patients, that appeared in *The American Journal of Clinical Nutrition*.

- Five percent of your body weight lost is the gold standard for proving the effectiveness of a weight-loss plan. But smoothie-based plans beat that number consistently. In a study at the University of Kentucky in 2009, patients were asked to drink at least three smoothies a day. After 18 weeks, the subjects lost an average of 16.4 percent of their body weight—up to 44 pounds!

- When researchers at Columbia University crunched the numbers on six separate studies following dieters on either a smoothie-based plan (one or two smoothies a day) or a reduced-calorie plan, they found that both sets lost weight, but those on the smoothie-based plan experienced "significantly greater weight loss" at both the three-month and one-year marks. In a 2015 review of studies on weight-loss plans, researchers at Johns Hopkins reported that participants who used low-calorie meal replacement drinks like smoothies lost more weight than other dieters over the course of four to six months.

Are you ready to make the magic work for you? You'll find a whole selection of life-changing shakes later in this book. There's something there to satisfy any craving.

LOSE YOUR BELLY RULE #4:
Double Down on Water

We want you to shoot for about 128 ounces of water a day, that's 16 eight-ounces glasses. (Remember that you get water from other beverages, such as coffee and tea, as well as the foods you eat; all count toward that quota.) Sound like a lot of trips to the bathroom? Maybe. But it's worth a little inconvenience. See, water fills your belly, curbing hunger. It's also essential for good digestion, and for your body to get the most out of the weight-loss nutrients like protein, healthy fats, flavonoids, and fiber. On the 7-Day Belly Melt Diet, it's crucial that you stay hydrated throughout the day. The reasons?

- Your body cannot efficiently change carbs into energy without ample water. And, according to the *Journal Physiology of Sport and Exercise*, you can't deliver essential amino acids to muscle tissue without adequate water, either. Not only will your muscles be undermined by dehydration, but insufficient liquids in your body will also hinder fat breakdown.

- Simply drinking more water may increase the rate at which healthy people burn calories, according to a study in *The Journal of Clinical Endocrinology and Metabolism*. After drinking approximately 17 ounces of water (about two tall glasses), participants' metabolic rates increased by 30 percent. The researchers estimate that increasing water intake by one-and-a half liters a day (about six cups) would burn an extra 17,400 calories over the course of the year—a weight loss of approximately five pounds!

- A study in the journal *Nature* found that drinking water unblocks fat-metabolizing mechanisms, perhaps because properly hydrated cells are better able to regulate fat metabolism. While simply drinking water throughout the day—especially when you first wake up, when your body is naturally dehydrated—will help keep your fat-burners on high, there's plenty of evidence that when you turn water into freshly brewed tea, it transforms into a true belly-shredding wonder. You've already read plenty in this book on the unique flavonoids found in tea, but later on, you'll discover even more ways that tea can help you strip off the pounds.

LOSE YOUR BELLY RULE #5:
Do the One Minute Morning Energizer

As we learned earlier, researchers at McMaster University determined that 60 seconds of intense exercise effort broken up into three 20-second chunks between longer segments of slow recovery exercise was the minimal exercise needed to reap health benefits. So we are going to use that minimalist approach to improve your aerobic fitness and health while you are on your way to becoming a more efficient calorie burner.

In the morning before you have your smoothie, find a spot in your home where you can move around a bit. Set your smartphone's stopwatch or use a clock with a minute hand. Do a two-minute warm-up: Begin by marching in place for 60 seconds at a slow pace. After that, do another minute of jumping jacks or seal jacks (instead of swinging arms overhead as in jumping jacks, swing them out to your sides every time you spread your legs; then, while jumping your feet back together, swing your parallel arm across your body and give your torso a bear hug). At the end of that second warm-up minute, do some sort of high-intensity exercise, such as speed walking, running, cycling or body-weight exercises like mountain climbers, push-ups, squat jumps, burpees, or lunges holding a full gallon water jug in front of your chest for resistance. In Chapter 11, we'll detail some options. Do your exercise of choice for 20 seconds as fast and intensely as possible. How do you know if you're pushing yourself hard enough? You quickly become breathless. You can do it. It's only for 20 seconds before you get to rest.

After 20 seconds, march in place, raising your knees high, almost to chest level, at a slow, recovery pace for one minute to catch your breath and recover from the intense effort. Follow that recovery minute with another 20 seconds of intense exercise and so on.

The workout will look like this:

- **Warm-up (two minutes)—60 seconds of a slow, steady march in place while circling your arms + 60 seconds of either jumping jacks or seal jacks**

- **High-intensity interval (20 seconds)— fast & hard total-body exercise**

- **Recovery (60 seconds)—slow, steady march in place**

- **High-intensity interval (20 seconds)— fast & hard total-body exercise**

- **Recovery (60 seconds)—slow, steady march in place**

- **High-intensity interval (20 seconds)— fast & hard total-body exercise**

- **Recovery (60 seconds). You're done!**

You've just completed one minute of intense exercise in an interval session of only six total minutes and reaped the health benefits of 45 minutes in the gym!

In Chapter 11, we'll show you variations of this morning workout involving various different types of cardio and body-weight exercises. Then, if you're inspired and ambitious, we'll show you how to do a simple strength workout using minimal equipment at home that'll help you build and tone calorie-burning lean muscle. The extra workout program will not only strengthen your biceps and tone your butt, it will do wonders for your heart health.

LOSE YOUR BELLY RULE #6:
Go to Bed by 10:30 Every Night

Getting enough sleep is one of the easiest ways to lose weight. Why? Because poor sleep habits pack on pounds. Studies show that when you are tired from inadequate rest, you are more likely to make poor eating decisions, gravitate toward processed carbohydrates, and consume larger portions and more calories overall. In fact, the Endocrine Society says missing out on even just 30 minutes of sleep a night can raise your risk of being overweight and developing diabetes. Second, lack of sleep decreases your production of leptin and increases ghrelin, reducing your ability to avoid tempting foods. And third, fatigue hampers insulin sensitivity, making it more difficult for your body to process the carbohydrates you eat.

Most experts suggest that seven to nine hours of quality sleep is what's ideal for most people. You'll need to determine how much makes you feel most rested and energetic in the morning. Try going to bed 15 minutes earlier than usual to see if that makes a difference. Figuring out your optimal sleep and getting it nightly can speed up belly melting: A study in the *American Journal of Clinical Nutrition* showed that well-rested subjects' resting energy expenditure—the amount of calories burned when a person isn't moving—was five percent higher than that of tired participants. The normal sleepers also burned 20 percent more calories after a meal versus sleep-deprived people.

9

Your 7-Day Belly Melt Meal Plan

Keep things simple; just follow this menu.

AS A KID, did you ever attempt to put a 1,000-piece puzzle together? Maybe Mom set up a card table in the corner of the den and left it there as you worked on it for weeks.

You either loved the meticulous challenge of hunting for the tiny pieces that fit into other tiny pieces or you felt it was too complicated, grew impatient, and quickly lost interest.

When you want to lose your belly rapidly, you can't mess with a 1,000-piece puzzle. Simplicity is critical. You want a plan that doesn't have a boxful of parts. It needs to be direct, minimal, and quick. And that's what you're getting here in this 7-day eating plan.

There are only four simple requirements to check off each day:

☑ Start each morning with a delicious, protein-rich breakfast smoothie.

☑ Focus on whole foods, versus processed ones, by following the F.L.A.V.O.R. foods guide.

☑ Make sure each main meal contains protein—that goes for most snacks, too.

☑ Drink water before and during each meal. We'd like to see you drinking up to 16 eight-ounce glasses of water a day. Unsweetened ice tea, hot tea, and coffee count toward that goal. The idea is to eliminate all beverage calories except for those you consume through smoothies. *

* This last rule is incredibly effective, especially if you regularly drink juice, soda, sweet tea, or alcoholic beverages.

Following these four simple requirements will magically whisk hundreds of calories from your daily diet.

How to Use This Meal Plan

Depending on what type of instruction follower you are, you can use this plan any number of ways. Some people like to be told exactly what to eat, when, and how much. Others find that prescription too restrictive. Some people, for example, simply won't eat calamari. Maybe you can't imagine eating kiwi because the fuzz gives you the heebie-jeebies. Maybe you want to keep things really, really simple and eat the same apple-and-peanut butter snack every morning at 10 and have the same grilled chicken salad for lunch every day. That's cool with us.

Feel free to follow this plan (you'll find it when you turn the page) to a T or use it as a general template into which you plug your personal preferences of foods or special recipes. As long as you follow those four general requirements and don't substitute in processed carbs or foods with added sugars, you are good to go. Flexibility is encouraged. Complicating things isn't.

Remember, to K.I.S.S. your belly good-bye, just **Keep It Simple, Sam.**

SAMPLE 7-DAY MEAL PLAN

Follow this menu or swap in other meals and snacks from recipes in Chapter 10.

DAY 1

BREAKFAST:
Chocolate Bean Smoothie (page 103)

SNACK 1:
Apple with peanut butter

LUNCH:
Baked Eggs with Mushrooms & Spinach (page 112)

SNACK 2:
Carrots and celery sticks with hummus

DINNER:
Herbed Roast Chicken with Root Vegetables (page 132)

DESSERT OR SNACK 3:
Mixed berries with whipped cream

DAY 2

BREAKFAST:
Kale 'n' Hearty Smoothie (page 105)

SNACK 1:
Fruit salad with oranges, blackberries, and cherries

LUNCH:
Minestrone with Pesto (page 113)

SNACK 2:
Yogurt with Pineapple, Kiwi, Mango, and Ginger Syrup (page 109)

DINNER:
Green Chile Cheeseburger (page 134) with Sweet Potato Fries (page 128) and Smoky Baked Beans (page 127)

DESSERT OR SNACK 3:
Cottage cheese with blueberries

DAY 3

BREAKFAST:
Walnut Mint Chip Smoothie (page 107)

SNACK 1:
Cottage cheese with blueberries or strawberries

LUNCH:
Hurry Up Hummus Soup (page 111)

SNACK 2:
1 hard-boiled egg

DINNER:
Classic Beef Stew (page 122)

DESSERT OR SNACK 3:
Yogurt with Pineapple, Kiwi, Mango, and Ginger Syrup, served as a parfait

DAY 4

BREAKFAST:
Cherry-Chocolate Tart Smoothie (page 104)

SNACK 1:
Plain Greek yogurt with fresh berries

LUNCH:
Grilled Calamari Salad (page 117)

SNACK 2:
Avocado half with salt, pepper, and lime

DINNER:
Roast Pork Loin with Lemony White Beans (page 133)

DESSERT OR SNACK 3:
Mixed berries with whipped cream

DAY 5

BREAKFAST:
Cantaloupe Kick Smoothie (page 103)

SNACK 1:
Cold rotisserie chicken pieces and red bell pepper slices

LUNCH:
Split Pea Soup (page 110)

SNACK 2:
Apple slices with Swiss cheese chunks

DINNER:
Bison Burger with Avocado (page 125)

DESSERT OR SNACK 3:
Mixed berries with whipped cream

DAY 6

BREAKFAST:
The Bluegrass Festival Smoothie (page 103)

SNACK 1:
Apple with 3 oz. hard cheese

LUNCH:
Greek Salad (page 116)

SNACK 2:
Whole unsalted almonds, small handful

DINNER:
Roast Salmon with Lentils (page 126)

DESSERT OR SNACK 3:
Yogurt with Pineapple, Kiwi, Mango, and Ginger Syrup, served as a parfait

DAY 7

BREAKFAST:
Cinnamon Girl Smoothie (page 102)

SNACK 1:
Baby carrots and hummus

LUNCH:
Fig & Prosciutto Salad (page 115)

SNACK 2:
Yogurt with Pineapple, Kiwi, Mango, and Ginger Syrup

DINNER:
Grilled Stuffed Portobello Mushrooms (page 136)

DESSERT OR SNACK 3:
Mixed berries with whipped cream

Belly Melt Diet Recipes

We give you lots of choices for delicious meals that will keep you healthy and satisfied.

THE MORE WE KNOW about the weight-loss power of flavonoids, the more it becomes clear that we need to squeeze fruits and vegetables into our day at every turn. If you filled out a food log at the start of the 7-Day Belly Melt Diet, review it. How many fruits and vegetables were you getting in a day? You see our point. These recipes are designed to pump up your diet with the fresh stuff while eliminating simple carbs and ensuring a healthy dose of fiber, protein, and fats.

The Belly Melt Breakfast

The American breakfast table is one of the hardest places to find flavonoids: Most traditional breakfasts are grains (cold cereal, oatmeal, doughnuts, English muffins, and the like), which we're going to be skipping for the next week, or they're eggs and bacon or maybe a cup of yogurt. Perhaps you squeeze in a fruit salad somewhere, but who wants to take the time to chop up fresh fruit—and worry about the leftovers—every morning?

That's why making a fruit-and-vegetable smoothie for breakfast each day is the easiest way to get a morning hit of flavonoids (plus protein, fiber, and healthy fats). It's the quickest, most delicious way to make up for the fruit-and-vegetable deficit: Roll out of bed, toss some produce in a blender, top with a bit of liquid, hit "liquefy." Boom! You're on the path to a skinnier, healthier existence.

Belly Melt Diet Smoothies

Making smoothies can be a pretty freewheeling endeavor, and that's certainly part of the fun, but we've established a few basic ground rules. Follow these and the ingredient-by-ingredient guide that follows and you'll be ready for your daily liquid flavonoids liftoff.

RULE #1: Always make sure you've got protein.
In most of the recipes that follow, you can use a protein powder. (We like vegan proteins because they eliminate the gassiness that whey can cause in those who are lactose intolerant.)

RULE #2: Play with your base. These recipes call for
almond milk, but a great way to sneak in additional flavonoids is to use green tea as your smoothie base. Green tea has been shown to be

extremely effective at attacking our fat-storage systems, and its mild taste makes for a pleasant base (unlike harsher black teas). Make a big pot of it and keep it chilling in your fridge for daily smoothie building.

RULE #3: Make sure you have fiber. To slow your digestion, keep you full, and ensure you're getting fiber daily, many of these recipes are made with fiber-rich fruits, and some even use beans. But you may also want to consider adding a fiber booster like psyllium husk or flaxmeal to make certain you're getting enough to reap all of its benefits.

RULE #4: Bring on the frozen fruit. Not only are they considerably more affordable, but research has found that frozen fruits may actually carry higher levels of flavonoids because they're picked at the height of their season and flash-frozen on the spot. Also, frozen fruit means you can use less ice to make your smoothie sufficiently cold, which in turn yields a more intense, pure flavor. (Make sure the fruit is unsweetened!)

RULE #5: Use a strong blender. A weak blender won't be able to crush the ice quickly enough, which means it melts and, ultimately, dilutes your precious creation, rather than giving it that bracingly chilled, velvety texture you want.

RULE #6: Respect the ratio. Once you learn the basic proportions of liquids to solids, you can turn anything into a pretty drinkable smoothie. The basic recipe: For every three cups of fruit, you'll need about one cup of base. Keep in mind that both yogurt and ice will thicken your drink.

Cinnamon Girl Smoothie

Studies have proven cinnamon's power as a blood sugar stabilizer. Adding a teaspoon of the spice to a carb-rich meal prevents insulin spikes that drive overeating, according to research in the *American Journal of Clinical Nutrition*. That makes this one heck of a belly-fat buster.

You'll Need

1   generous handful of collard greens
1   pear, chopped
1   medium apple, chopped
1   tsp. cinnamon
1   Tbsp. plant-based protein powder
1   cup water
1   cup ice

Makes 2 servings

Per serving: 150 calories, 1 g fat, 32 g carbohydrates, 12 g fiber, 6 g protein

Cantaloupe Kick Smoothie

A great combination of flavors inspired by Mexican cuisine. Just ½ teaspoon of hot pepper can help reduce appetite after a meal, according to a study at Purdue University. And daily consumption of capsaicin, the active ingredient in cayenne, speeds abdominal weight loss, according to a study in the *American Journal of Clinical Nutrition*.

You'll Need

1   cup cantaloupe
½   cup mango
1   dash cayenne pepper
1   cup unsweetened almond milk
1   Tbsp. ground chia seeds
⅓   cup chocolate plant-based protein powder
6   cubes ice
Water to blend (optional)

Makes 2 servings

Per serving: 298 calories, 5 g fat, 35 g carbs, 6 g fiber, 29 g protein

Chocolate Bean Smoothie

Beans? In a smoothie? Use canned or precooked beans for a thick, earthy protein and fiber punch. One study found that people who ate ¾ cup of beans daily weighed 6.6 pounds less, on average, than those who didn't, even though the bean eaters took in more calories.

You'll Need
½   frozen banana
¼   cup black beans
1   teaspoon nutmeg
1   cup unsweetened almond milk
⅓   cup chocolate plant-based protein powder
Water to blend (optional)

Makes 1 serving

Per serving: 280 calories, 3 g fat, 31 g carbohydrates, 7 g fiber, 31 g protein

The Bluegrass Festival Smoothie

Blueberries, spinach, and avocado all in one dish? It's like an Avengers movie. And sure enough, it's super! The fat in the avocados helps make the folate and flavonoids in the spinach and berries more bioavailable. Studies show that women who eat foods with high water content, such as spinach, have a lower BMI (Body Mass Index) and smaller waistlines than those who don't.

You'll Need
¼   cup blueberries
1   cup spinach, chopped
¼   avocado, peeled and pitted
½   cup unsweetened almond milk
1   scoop vanilla plant-based protein powder
Water to blend (optional)

Makes 1 serving

Per serving: 292 calories, 12 g fat, 18 g carbohydrates, 7 g fiber, 29 g protein

Cherry-Chocolate Tart Smoothie

We feel cherries and bananas don't spend nearly as much time together as they ought to, and you'll agree with us after you taste this. Using banana gives you an extra hit of resistant starch, a type of carbohydrate that slows digestion and helps make your belly biome stronger, according to a 2015 study in the *Journal of Functional Foods*.

You'll Need
½ banana
½ cup cherries, pitted
1 Tbsp. unsweetened cocoa powder
Dash of nutmeg
¼ cup black beans
½ cup unsweetened almond milk
¼ cup chocolate plant-based protein powder
6 ice cubes
Water to blend (optional)

Makes 1 serving

Per serving: 294 calories, 2 g fat, 41 g carbohydrates, 11 g fiber, 25 g protein

Back in Black Smoothie

This smoothie combines the powers of citrus, green vegetables, and dark berries to keep your body's flavonoid funds "in the black."

You'll Need
½ cup frozen blackberries
Juice of ½ lemon
1 cup spinach
1 cup unsweetened almond milk
1 scoop plain or flavored plant-based protein powder

Makes 1 serving

Per serving: 219 calories, 4.7 g fat, 18.5 g carbohydrates, 8 g fiber, 28 g protein

Fruit Loopers Smoothie

The fiber from the chia seeds and good fats from avocado will keep blood sugar stable despite all the fruit crammed into this shake.

You'll Need

½   frozen banana
1   medium apple, cored and chopped
1   scoop whey protein powder
½   avocado
½   cup strawberries, sliced
1   tsp. chia seeds
½   tsp. grated fresh ginger
½   cup coconut milk

Makes 2 servings

Per serving: 300 calories, 15 g fat, 26 g carbohydrates, 12 g fiber, 10 g protein

Kale 'n' Hearty Smoothie

Want to keep your belly biome happy? To make sure your gut is in good shape, you need to feed your abdominal allies something called fructooligosaccharides, or FOS, a type of fiber found in fruits and leafy greens. This drink will get the party started and help heal your gut while enticing your taste buds.

You'll Need

1   cup kale
½   cup chopped cucumber, peeled and seeded
½   pear, seeded and quartered
Squeeze of fresh lime juice
1   scoop plain or vanilla plant-based protein powder
½   cup water
2   ice cubes

Makes 1 serving

Per serving: 217 calories, 1 g fat, 26 g carbohydrates, 5 g fiber, 28 g protein

Chicory–Root Beer Smoothie

Add chicory to the list of overlooked fat fighters. More nutritious than lettuce or even kale, chicory is the primary source of inulin, the soluble fiber that's added to products like Activia to promote a healthy belly biome.

You'll Need

½   cup chicory
½   cup spinach
¼   apple with peel, seeded and quartered
½   frozen banana
1   tsp. chia seeds
1   cup water
1   scoop plain plant-based protein powder
Touch of honey
Water to blend (optional)*
*   After blending, add a splash of soda water for fizz.

Makes 1 serving

Per serving: 231 calories, 2 g fat, 27 g carbohydrates, 5.5 g fiber, 28 g protein

---

The Strawvocado Smoothie

It may not look, act, or taste like it, but the avocado is a fruit (so are olives). When you add avocado to a smoothie, you give it a big boost of belly-satisfying monounsaturated fats. Note: Avocado will dramatically reduce your appetite for up to four hours. Deploy accordingly.

You'll Need

¼   avocado, peeled, pitted, and quartered
½   cup frozen strawberries
½   cup unsweetened almond milk
1   scoop plain or vanilla plant-based protein powder
Squeeze of fresh lemon juice
2   ice cubes
Water to blend (optional)

Makes 1 serving

Per serving: 289 calories, 12 g fat, 18 g carbohydrates, 7 g fiber, 28 g protein

Walnut Mint Chip Smoothie

Walnuts' fiber and fat combine to make you feel fuller longer, making them one of the best weight-loss foods. One review of 31 clinical trials found that study participants whose diets included walnuts lost about 1.4 extra pounds and half an inch from their waists.

You'll Need

¼   cup walnuts
½   cup unsweetened almond milk
1   medium banana, greenish skin, not quite ripe
¾   cup baby spinach
¼   cup fresh mint leaves
½   tsp. peppermint oil
4   ice cubes
1   Tbsp. cacao nibs to garnish
½   cup water (if it's too thick for you)

- Save a few mint leaves and some cacao nibs for a garnish, then put the rest of the ingredients in a powerful blender and blend until smooth. Add water if too thick.

Makes 1 serving

Per serving: 350 calories, 27 g fat, 22 g carbohydrates, 7 g fiber, 7 g protein

Belly Melt Diet Lunches

By the time lunch rolls around, you've already had a filling breakfast, then you topped it off with a nice snack of fruits and/or vegetables. So you might not feel particularly hungry. That's fine. To stay within the Diet's rules, look for salads with nice pieces of protein, or opt for chunky soups with vegetables and meat. Avoid salad dressings unless you know what's in them; most are sugar-water with a little bit of oil mixed in. Instead, ask for oil and vinegar on the side, and mix it yourself, finishing it with some salt and pepper.

Smoked Salmon "Sandwich"

You'll Need

¼	cup whipped cream cheese
8	large whole-grain crackers*
2	Tbsp. capers, rinsed and chopped
½	red onion, thinly sliced
2	cups mixed baby greens
1	small tomato, sliced
Salt and black pepper, to taste	
8	oz. smoked salmon
*	These can be made with toasted bread after completing the 7-Day Belly Melt Diet when you have moved to the maintenance portion of the diet.

How to Make It

- Spread 1 tablespoon of the cream cheese on each of the crackers. Top each with capers, onion, greens, and a slice of tomato. Lightly salt the tomato, then add as much pepper as you'd like (this sandwich cries out for a lot of it). Finish by draping a few slices of smoked salmon over the tomatoes and topping with the remaining crackers.

Makes 4 sandwiches

Per serving: 238 calories, 7 g fat (3 g saturated), 18 g carbohydrates, 4 g fiber, 12 g sugars, 17 g protein

Yogurt with Pineapple, Kiwi, Mango, and Ginger Syrup

You'll Need

1	cup water
¼	cup sugar
1	-in. piece peeled fresh ginger, sliced
24	oz. Greek-style yogurt (four 6-oz. containers)
2	kiwis, peeled and sliced
1	cup chopped pineapple
1	mango, peeled, pitted, and chopped
½	cup granola (optional)*

* The granola is added for texture, but use it sparingly even after you've finished the 7 days of the Belly Melt Diet and add it back into your diet: Those little clusters are dense with calories.

How to Make It

- **For the syrup:** Combine the water, sugar, and ginger in a small saucepan and bring to a boil. Simmer for 10 minutes. Let cool for at least 10 minutes. Discard the ginger pieces.

- **For the yogurt:** Divide the yogurt among four bowls, top with the fruits and granola, then drizzle with the ginger syrup. For a more dramatic presentation, layer the yogurt, fruit, granola, and syrup in tall glasses, like parfaits.

Makes 4 servings

Per serving: 321 calories, 6 g fat (3 g saturated), 57 g carbohydrates, 4 g fiber, 47 g sugars, 15 g protein

Asparagus with Fried Eggs and Prosciutto

You'll Need

1 bunch asparagus, woody ends removed

3 Tbsp. olive oil, divided

4 large eggs

4 slices prosciutto, cut into thin strips

2 Tbsp. vinegar

Coarse sea salt and black pepper, to taste

How to Make It

- For the asparagus: Bring a large pot of water to a boil and season with a healthy pinch of salt. Add the asparagus and cook for 3 to 4 minutes, until just tender. Drain and run under cold water to stop the cooking process (which will also help preserve asparagus color).

- Heat 1 tablespoon of the oil in a large nonstick sauté pan. Crack the eggs into the pan and cook for about 5 minutes, just until the whites are set but the yolks are still loose.

- Divide the asparagus among 4 plates. Top each serving with a fried egg and the prosciutto strips. Drizzle with the remaining olive oil and the vinegar and season with salt and black pepper.

Makes 4 servings

Per serving: 277 calories, 20 g fat (4 g saturated), 10 g carbohydrates, 2 g fiber, 2 g sugars, 17 g protein

Split Pea Soup

You'll Need

1 tsp. olive oil

2 ribs celery, diced

1 small onion, diced

2 medium carrots, peeled and diced

2 cloves garlic, minced

10 cups water or low-sodium chicken or vegetable stock

2 medium red potatoes, peeled and diced

1 smoked ham hock

1 cup split peas

2 bay leaves

Salt and black pepper, to taste

Tabasco, to taste (optional)

How to Make It

- Heat the olive oil in a large saucepan or pot over medium heat. Add the celery, onion, carrots, and garlic and sauté for about 5 minutes, until the vegetables are soft. Add the water or stock, the potatoes, ham hock, split peas, and bay leaves. Turn the heat down to low and simmer for about 40 minutes, until the peas have turned very soft and begin to lose their shape, leaving you with a thick soup. (Thin out with more water or stock if you prefer a thinner consistency.)

- Remove the ham hock, shred the meat clinging to the bone, and add the meat back to the soup. Discard the bay leaves. Season to taste with salt and pepper, plus a few shakes of Tabasco, if you like.

Makes 6 servings

Per serving: 234 calories, 11 g fat (3 g saturated), 23 g carbohydrates, 4 g fiber, 3 g sugars, 11 g protein

---

Hurry-Up Hummus Soup

You'll Need

2   (10-oz.) containers spicy hummus
4   cups reduced-sodium chicken or vegetable broth
1   (15-oz.) can chickpeas, drained
1   (12-oz.) jar roasted red peppers, drained and chopped
⅔   cup pitted Kalamata olives, chopped
⅓   cup chopped flat-leaf parsley, plus a bit extra for garnish
2   Tbsp. extra-virgin olive oil, divided

How to Make It

- Place hummus, reduced-sodium chicken or vegetable broth, chickpeas, red peppers, Kalamata olives, and leaf parsley into a 6-quart saucepan. Bring to a simmer over medium heat and continue to cook for 10 to 15 minutes.

- Divide among 6 bowls and drizzle with 1 teaspoon of olive oil and a few flecks of parsley for garnish.

Makes 6 servings

Per serving: 482 calories, 24 g fat (3 g saturated), 54 g carbohydrates, 14 g fiber, 9 g sugars, 18 g protein

Baked Eggs with Mushrooms and Spinach

You'll Need

1	Tbsp. olive oil
1	small onion, chopped
2	cups mushrooms, sliced
4	slices Canadian bacon or deli ham, cut into thin strips
½	(10-oz.) bag frozen spinach, thawed
½	(7-oz.) can roasted green chiles

Salt and black pepper, to taste

4   eggs

How to Make It

- Preheat the oven to 375°F. Heat the oil in a large skillet set over medium heat. Add the onion and cook for about 3 minutes, until translucent. Add the mushrooms and cook for about 5 minutes, until lightly browned. Stir in the bacon, spinach, and chiles and cook for a few minutes, until the spinach is heated through. If any water from the spinach accumulates in the pan, carefully drain. Season with salt and pepper.

- Divide the mixture among four 6-ounce oven-safe ramekins that have been lightly greased with butter. Carefully crack an egg into each, making sure to keep the yolks intact. Place the ramekins in a baking dish and bake until the whites are just set but the yolks are still runny, about 10 minutes.

Makes 4 servings

Per serving: 169 calories, 9 g fat (3 g saturated), 6 g carbohydrates, 1 g fiber, 3 g sugars, 15 g protein

Minestrone with Pesto

You'll Need

1	Tbsp. olive oil
1	medium onion, chopped
2	cloves garlic, minced
8	oz. Yukon gold or red potatoes, cubed
2	medium carrots, peeled and chopped
1	medium zucchini, chopped
8	oz. green beans, ends trimmed, halved

Salt and black pepper, to taste

1	(14-oz.) can diced tomatoes
8	cups low-sodium chicken stock (or a mixture of stock and water)
½	tsp. dried thyme
½	(14–16-oz.) can white beans (aka cannellini), drained

Pesto

Parmesan, for grating

How to Make It

- Heat the olive oil in a large pot over medium heat. Add the onion and garlic and cook until the onion is translucent, about 3 minutes. Stir in the potatoes, carrots, zucchini, and green beans. Season with a bit of salt and cook, stirring, for 3 to 4 minutes to release the vegetables' aromas. Add the tomatoes, stock, and thyme and turn the heat down to low. Season with salt (if still needed) and pepper to taste. Simmer for at least 15 minutes, and up to 45.

- Before serving, stir in the white beans and heat through. Serve with a dollop of pesto and bit of grated Parmesan.

Makes 4 servings

Per serving: 383 calories, 14 g fat (3 g saturated), 53 g carbohydrates, 11 g fiber, 8 g sugars, 19 g protein

Avocado-Crab Salad

You'll Need

1   (8-oz.) can crabmeat, preferably jumbo lump,* drained
½   cup diced, seeded, and peeled cucumber
¼   cup minced red onion
¼   cup chopped cilantro
1   jalapeño pepper (preferably red), minced
1   Tbsp. fish sauce (in a pinch, soy sauce will do)
1   Tbsp. sugar
Juice of 1 lime
Salt
4   small Hass avocados, halved and pitted
1   lime, quartered
*   Jumbo lump gives you the largest, sweetest hunks of crab, but it also
    comes with the steepest price tag. Backfin crab is a more affordable
    variety made from broken-up lumps.

How to Make It

- Combine the crab, cucumber, onion, cilantro, jalapeño, fish sauce,
  sugar, and lime juice in a mixing bowl. Stir gently to combine, being
  careful not to break up the bigger lumps of crab.

- Lightly salt the flesh of the avocados, then divide the crab mixture
  among the 8 halves, spooning it directly into the bowls created by
  removing the pits. Serve with the lime quarters.

Makes 4 servings

Per serving: 152 calories, 8 g fat (1 g saturated), 11 g carbohydrates,
4 g fiber, 7 g sugars, 11 g protein

Fig & Prosciutto Salad

You'll Need

¼   cup pine nuts, toasted

12   cups baby arugula

8   figs (preferably Mission)*

6   slices prosciutto, cut into thin strips

½   cup crumbled fresh goat cheese

Salt and black pepper, to taste

2   Tbsp. minced shallots (about 2 small)

1   garlic clove, minced

2   tsp. Dijon mustard

¼   cup balsamic vinegar

½   cup olive oil

*   Can't find figs at the local market? Sliced ripe peaches or strawberries make an excellent substitute.

How to Make It

- The Balsamic Vinaigrette dressing: Combine the shallots, garlic, Dijon, and balsamic in a large mixing bowl, along with a good pinch of salt and pepper. Slowly drizzle in the olive oil, whisking as you do. Alternatively, you can combine all the ingredients in a clean mason jar and shake like crazy for 20 seconds. Keeps for 1 week covered in the refrigerator.

- For the salad: Toast the nuts by spreading them on a baking sheet and baking in a 375°F oven for about 10 minutes.

- Combine the arugula, figs, prosciutto, pine nuts, and goat cheese in a large salad bowl, along with a few pinches of salt and plenty of black pepper. Pour in just enough of the homemade Balsamic Vinaigrette to cling lightly to the lettuce and toss gently. Divide among 4 plates.

Makes 4 servings

Per serving with dressing: 415 calories, 29 g fat (5 g saturated), 29 g carbohydrates, 5 g fiber, 24 g sugars, 18 g protein

Greek Salad

You'll Need

2   cups shredded or chopped cooked chicken*
1   large cucumber, peeled, seeded, and chopped
1   red bell pepper, chopped
4   Roma tomatoes, chopped
1   red onion, chopped
½   (14–16-oz.) can garbanzo beans, drained
¾   cup crumbled feta
2   Tbsp. red wine vinegar
1   tsp. dried oregano
Salt and black pepper, to taste
¼   cup olive oil
*   This salad would be just as good made with canned tuna, chopped hard-boiled egg, or no main protein at all.

How to Make It

- Combine the chicken, cucumber, bell pepper, tomato, onion, beans, and feta in a large salad bowl. In a separate bowl, combine the vinegar and oregano with a few generous pinches of salt and pepper. Slowly drizzle in the olive oil, tossing to combine.

- You can serve now, but it's best to let this one sit in the fridge for 30 minutes or so, which gives all the ingredients a chance to get friendly.

Makes 4 servings

Per serving: 336 calories, 25 g fat (2 g saturated), 21 g carbohydrates, 6 g fiber, 3 g sugars, 20 g protein

Grilled Calamari Salad

You'll Need

1   lb. squid, cleaned, tentacles reserved for another use
½   Tbsp. peanut or canola oil
Salt and black pepper, to taste
Juice of 1 lime
1   Tbsp. fish sauce
1   Tbsp. sugar
½   Tbsp. chili garlic sauce (preferably sambal oelek)
4   cups watercress*
1   small cucumber, peeled, seeded, and cut into matchsticks
1   medium tomato, chopped
½   red onion, very thinly sliced
¼   cup roasted peanuts
*   Watercress isn't always easy to find. Baby arugula, or even a few big
     handfuls of fresh basil leaves, can easily take its place here.

How to Make It

- Preheat a grill. Toss the squid bodies with the oil and generously
  season with salt and lots of black pepper. When the grill is very hot,
  add the squid and grill for about 5 minutes, until lightly charred all
  over.

- Combine the lime juice, fish sauce, sugar, and chili sauce in a mixing
  bowl and whisk to blend. Slice the grilled squid into ½-inch rings. In a
  salad bowl, toss the squid, watercress, cucumber, tomato, onion, and
  peanuts with the dressing. Divide the salad among 4 plates.

Makes 4 servings

Per serving with dressing: 143 calories, 3 g fat (1 g saturated),
9 g carbohydrates, 0 g fiber, 4 g sugars, 18 g protein

Chicken & White Bean Chili

You'll Need

1	Tbsp. olive oil
2	yellow onions, chopped
4	cloves garlic, minced
1	lb. boneless, skinless chicken thighs, cut into small pieces*
1	lb. lean ground chicken
1	(7-oz.) can roasted green chiles
1	tsp. ground cumin
1	tsp. dried oregano
¼	tsp. cayenne pepper
4	cups low-sodium chicken stock
2	(14–16-oz.) cans white kidney beans (also called cannellini and great Northern beans), drained

Salt and black pepper, to taste

Fresh cilantro, shredded cheese, diced onion, sour cream, and/or sliced jalapeños, for serving

* The mix of ground and chopped chicken gives this chili a more interesting texture, but if you prefer one over the other, simply use 2 pounds of your chicken of choice.

Roasting Peppers

A simple heating process gives peppers a smoky sweetness that can enhance lots of savory dishes.

You can buy bottled roasted red peppers in any supermarket, but save a few bucks and roast them yourself instead. Cook the bell peppers (red and yellow are best) at 400°F until the skin blackens and the flesh softens, about 25 minutes (you can also do this on a grill or even over a low flame on a gas stovetop). Remove peppers from heat, then place in a bowl, cover with plastic wrap, and let sit for 10 minutes. Remove the plastic wrap and peel off the dark skin (the steam created by covering the peppers makes this easy). Discard the stems and seeds, and they're ready to eat.

How to Make It

• Heat the oil in a large pot over medium heat. Add the onion and garlic and cook for about 3 minutes, until the onion is translucent. Add the chicken thighs, ground chicken, chiles, cumin, oregano, and cayenne. Sauté until the chicken is mostly cooked through, about 8 minutes. Add the stock and beans. Turn the heat down to low.

• Simmer uncovered for at least 20 minutes, or longer if you have the patience. Taste the chili and adjust the seasoning with salt and pepper. Serve with any combination of the garnishes.

Makes 8 servings

Per serving (without toppings): 226 calories, 9 g fat, (2 g saturated), 13 g carbohydrates, 5 g fiber, 1 g sugars, 27 g protein

---

Grilled Chicken with Chimichurri

You'll Need

1 cup rough-chopped parsley (about half a bunch)
1 clove garlic
½ tsp. salt
2 Tbsp. water
1½ Tbsp. red wine vinegar
¼ cup oil
½ tsp. sugar
1 Tbsp. minced jalapeño
4 boneless skinless chicken thighs (6 oz. each)*
Salt and black pepper, to taste
2 cups mixed baby greens
½ red onion, thinly sliced
½ cup jarred roasted red peppers
* Want to save yourself the trouble of cooking the chicken? Use the meat from a store-bought rotisserie bird instead.

How to Make It

• For the chimichurri: Combine parsley, garlic, salt, water, red wine vinegar, oil, sugar, and jalapeño in a food processor and pulse until fully blended. Keeps in the refrigerator for up to one week.

• For the chicken: Preheat a grill, grill pan, or cast-iron skillet. Season the chicken all over with salt and pepper and grill or sear for 3 to 4 minutes per side, until firm and cooked through.

- Divide the mixed greens among plates. Top each plate with a chicken thigh, then pile on the onion and peppers. Spoon about ½ cup chimichurri on top.

Makes 4 servings

Per serving: 298 calories, 11 g fat (2 g saturated), 19 g carbohydrates, 1 g fiber, 2 g sugars, 22 g protein

---

Spinach and Goat Cheese Salad with Apples and Warm Bacon Dressing

You'll Need

6	strips bacon, chopped
1	small red onion, sliced
1	green apple, peeled and sliced
¼	cup pecans
2	Tbsp. red wine vinegar
1	Tbsp. Dijon Mustard
1	Tbsp. olive oil
1	bunch spinach, washed, dried, and stemmed
¼	cup fresh goat cheese

Salt and black pepper, to taste

How to Make It

- Heat a large cast-iron skillet or nonstick pan over medium heat. Add the bacon and cook for about 5 minutes, until browned and just crisp. Remove to a paper towel-lined plate and reserve.

- Add the onion to the same pan and cook for 2 to 3 minutes, until just soft. Add the apple and pecans and continue sautéing for 2 minutes, until the pecans are lightly toasted and the apple softened. Add the vinegar, mustard, and olive oil, along with a few pinches of salt and plenty of black pepper. Use a wooden spoon to stir the mixture vigorously to help it emulsify into a unified dressing.

- Divide the spinach and goat cheese among 4 bowls and pour the warm dressing directly over the greens. Garnish with the reserved bacon.

Makes 4 servings

Per serving: 201 calories, 14 g fat (3 saturated), 13 g carbohydrates, 4 g fiber, 6 g sugars, 8 g protein

Chinese Chicken Salad

You'll Need

1   head napa cabbage

½   head red cabbage

½   Tbsp. sugar

2   cups chopped or shredded cooked chicken (freshly grilled or from a store-bought rotisserie chicken)

⅓   cup Asian-style dressing, like Annie's Shiitake and Sesame Vinaigrette

1   cup fresh cilantro leaves

1   cup canned mandarin oranges (stored in water), drained

¼   cup sliced almonds, toasted

Salt and black pepper, to taste

How to Make It

- Cut the cabbage heads in half lengthwise and remove the cores. Slice the cabbage into thin strips. Toss with the sugar in a large bowl.

- If the chicken is cold, toss a few tablespoons of vinaigrette and heat in microwave at 50 percent power. Add to the cabbage, along with the cilantro, mandarins, almonds, and the remaining vinaigrette. Toss to combine. Season with salt and pepper.

Makes 4 servings

Per serving: 355 calories, 21 g fat (3 g saturated), 21 g carbohydrates, 4 g fiber, 15 g sugars, 22 g protein

Belly Melt Diet Dinners

At least half the time we sit down to eat dinner, we're celebrating something. We're with friends, we're with family, the game is on—something's usually happening that makes dinner different from other meals. That's why dinner is when we most often fall off of our diet plans.

Fortunately, the Belly Melt Diet rules are pretty easy to follow at dinnertime: Avoid pastas, bread, rice, and other grains, and look for lean meats and plenty of vegetables. Try to have beans or legumes at least a few times a week; fish a couple of times a week; poultry once or twice a week. That leaves a couple of days for your favorite red meat. And as always, make sure ¾ of your bowl or plate is produce.

Classic Beef Stew

You'll Need

2   Tbsp. minced garlic (optional)
½   cup minced fresh parsley (optional)
1   Tbsp. grated lemon zest (optional)
1   Tbsp. canola oil, divided
3   lb. sirloin roast, brisket, or chuck, cut into 1-in. cubes
1   Tbsp. flour
Salt and black pepper, to taste
2   medium onions, chopped
1   cup dry red wine, such as Pinot Noir or Cabernet Sauvignon
2   Tbsp. tomato paste
2   cups chicken broth
3   bay leaves
8   branches fresh thyme (or 1 tsp. dried)
6   medium red potatoes, cut into ½-in. pieces
3   medium carrots, peeled and chopped
2   cups frozen pearl onions
1   cup frozen peas

How to Make It

- For the gremolata (optional): Combine the garlic with the parsley and lemon zest. Set aside.

- For the stew: Heat ½ tablespoon of the oil in a large cast-iron skillet or sauté pan over medium-high heat. Combine the beef and flour in a bowl, season with salt and pepper, and toss to lightly coat the beef. Working in two batches to avoid crowding the pan, sear the beef in the hot oil, turning occasionally until nicely browned. Transfer to a slow cooker.

- Add the remaining oil to the skillet. Add the chopped onions and cook for about 5 minutes, until lightly browned. Stir in the wine and tomato paste, scraping the bottom of the pan to free up any browned bits. Pour the onion mixture over the beef, then add the broth, bay leaves, and thyme. Set the slow cooker to high, cover, and cook for about 4 hours (or on low for 8 hours), until the beef is fork-tender.

- An hour before serving, add the potatoes, carrots, and pearl onions. Five minutes before serving, add the peas. Discard the bay leaves and thyme branches and season with salt and black pepper. Serve garnished with parsley or the gremolata (optional).

Makes 8 servings

Per serving: 400 calories, 10 g fat (3 g saturated), 33 g carbohydrates, 5 g fiber, 7 g sugars, 36 g protein

Shrimp Scampi

You'll Need

1   Tbsp. olive oil
3   cloves garlic, minced
Red pepper flakes
1   small red onion, thinly sliced
1   lb. medium shrimp, peeled and deveined
Salt and black pepper, to taste
Chopped flat-leaf parsley
Zest and juice from 1 lemon

How to Make It

- Heat the olive oil in a large skillet or sauté pan over medium heat. Add the garlic and pepper flakes and cook until the garlic is light brown. Add the onion and continue cooking until it is translucent.

- Season the shrimp with a pinch of salt and add to the pan. Cook, stirring occasionally, until the shrimp are pink and lightly caramelized. Remove from the heat, stir in the parsley, lemon zest, and lemon juice. Season with salt and pepper. Serve as is or on top of a small portion of buttered chickpea pasta or quinoa.

Makes 4 servings

Per serving: 123 calories, 4 g fat (0 g saturated), 7 g carbohydrates, 2 g fiber, 1 g sugars, 29 g protein

Grilled Chicken Salad

You'll Need

½   Tbsp. honey
1   Tbsp. Dijon mustard
2   Tbsp. red or white wine vinegar
¼   cup canola oil
Salt and black pepper, to taste
12   oz. cooked chicken
12   cups arugula (1 prewashed bag)
¼   cup dried cranberries
1   avocado, pitted, peeled, and sliced
¼   cup crumbled goat cheese
¼   cup walnuts, roughly chopped

How to Make It

● For the Honey-Mustard Vinaigrette: Combine honey, Dijon mustard, red or white wine vinegar, canola oil, and salt and pepper. Set aside.

● For the salad: Combine the chicken, arugula, cranberries, avocado, goat cheese, and walnuts. Top with ¼ cup of the vinaigrette, salt, and pepper in a large bowl, using your hands or two forks to fully incorporate the dressing before serving.

Makes 4 servings

Per serving: 296 calories, 20 g fat (2 g saturated), 15 g carbohydrates, 4 g fiber, 9 g sugars, 20 g protein

---

Bunless Bison Burger with Avocado

You'll Need

1½ lb. ground grass-fed bison
1 tsp. lime juice
Salt and pepper
1 large avocado
Havarti cheese slices
Handful of arugula

How to Make It

● Add lime juice to the ground bison in a bowl and mix. Form into 4 equal patties and season with salt and pepper. Cook patties on a grill or in a grill pan over medium heat. Cook for 4 to 6 minutes on each side. Be careful not to overcook. Use a thermometer and cook to an internal temperature of 160°F.

● While the bison is cooking, peel and pit an avocado, quarter it, and slice each quarter.

● About a minute and a half before the burgers are done, top each patty with a slice of Havarti cheese; let it melt. Take the patties off the grill and allow to rest on a plate for a few minutes to let the juice reabsorb.

● Divide the arugula leaves on four plates. Place a burger on top of each pile of arugula and top with the avocado slices.

Makes 4 servings

Per serving: 418 calories, 22 g fat (7 g saturated), 20 g carbohydrates, 2 g fiber, 3 g sugars, 49 g protein

Roast Salmon with Lentils

You'll Need

½   Tbsp. olive oil
1   medium carrot, peeled and diced
½   medium yellow onion, diced
2   cloves garlic, minced
1   cup dried lentils
3   cups chicken broth or water
2   bay leaves
2   Tbsp. red wine vinegar
Salt and black pepper, to taste
4   salmon fillets (4 oz. each)
2   Tbsp. Dijon mustard
2   Tbsp. brown sugar

How to Make It

- Preheat the oven to 450°F.

- Heat the olive oil in a medium saucepan over medium heat. Add the carrot, onion, and garlic and sauté for 5 to 7 minutes, until soft and lightly browned. Add the lentils, broth, and bay leaves. Simmer for about 20 minutes, until the lentils are tender and the liquid has mostly evaporated. Before serving, add the vinegar, season with salt and pepper, and discard the bay leaves.

- While the lentils simmer, roast the salmon: Season the fish with salt and black pepper. Combine the mustard and brown sugar in a mixing bowl and spread evenly over the salmon fillets.

- Place the salmon on a baking sheet and place on the top rack of the oven. Roast for 8 to 10 minutes, until the salmon has browned on the surface and flakes with gentle pressure from your finger.

- Divide the lentils among 4 plates or pasta bowls and top each serving with a piece of salmon.

Makes 4 servings

Per serving: 375 calories, 11 g fat (0 g saturated fat), 24 g carbohydrates, 3 g fiber, 8 g sugars, 38 g protein

Smoky Baked Beans

You'll Need
4   strips bacon, chopped into small pieces
1   medium onion, minced
2   cloves garlic, minced
2   (16-oz.) cans pinto beans, rinsed and drained
1   cup dark beer
¼   cup ketchup
1   Tbsp. chili powder
1   Tbsp. brown sugar
Pinch of cayenne pepper

How to Make It
- Heat a large pot or saucepan over medium heat. Add the bacon and cook until it's just turning crispy, 3 to 5 minutes.

- Add the onion and garlic and sauté until translucent, another 3 minutes.

- Stir in the beans, beer, ketchup, chili powder, brown sugar, and cayenne. Simmer until the sauce thickens and clings to the beans, about 15 minutes.

Makes 6 servings

Per serving: 266 calories, 4 g fat (1 g saturated), 30 g carbohydrates, 8 g fiber, 3 g sugars, 10 g protein

Sweet Potato Fries

You'll Need
2   medium sweet potatoes, peeled and cut into wedges
1   Tbsp. olive oil
Pinch of cayenne
½   tsp. smoked paprika (optional)
Salt and black pepper, to taste

How to Make It
- Preheat the oven to 425°F. Combine all the ingredients, plus a generous amount of salt and pepper, on a baking sheet and toss to coat evenly. Bake until the sweet potatoes have browned on the outside, are crisp to the touch, and are tender inside, about 25 minutes.

Makes 4 servings

Per serving: 87 calories, 3 g fat (0 g saturated), 13 g carbohydrates, 2 g fiber, 3 g sugars, 1 g protein

---

Grilled Mahi Mahi with Red Pepper Sauce

You'll Need
¾   cup chopped fresh parsley
¼   cup chopped fresh mint (optional)
Juice of 1 lemon
¼   cup olive oil, plus more for grilling
2-3 anchovy fillets, minced
2   Tbsp. capers, rinsed and chopped
1   clove garlic, crushed
Pinch of red pepper flakes
Salt and black pepper, to taste
4   mahi mahi fillets, or other firm white fish like halibut, sea bass, or swordfish (about 6 oz. each)

How to Make It
- Preheat a grill. Make sure the grate is cleaned and oiled.

- For the Red Pepper Sauce: Combine the parsley, mint if using, lemon juice, olive oil, anchovies, capers, garlic, and pepper flakes in a mixing bowl. Season with black pepper. Set aside.

- **For the fish:** Rub the fish with a thin layer of oil, then season all over with salt and pepper. Place the fillets on the grill skin side down and grill for 5 minutes, until the skin is lightly charred and crisp and pulls away freely (if you mess with the fish before it's read to flip, it's likely to stick). Flip and cook on the other side for 2 to 3 minutes longer, until the fish flakes with gentle pressure from your fingertip. Serve the fillets with the Red Pepper Sauce spooned over the top.

Makes 4 servings

Per serving: 279 calories, 15 g fat (2 g saturated), 3 g carbohydrates, 1 g fiber, 1 g sugars, 32 g protein

---

Garlic-Lemon Spinach

You'll Need

1   Tbsp. olive oil
3   cloves garlic, thinly sliced
Pinch red pepper flakes
2   bunches spinach, stems removed, washed, and dried
Juice of 1 lemon
Salt and black pepper, to taste

How to Make It

- Heat the olive oil in a large sauté or saucepan over medium-low heat. Add the garlic and red pepper flakes and cook gently for about 3 minutes, until the garlic is lightly browned.

- Add the spinach and cook, moving the uncooked spinach to the bottom of the pan with tongs, for about 5 minutes, until fully wilted. Drain off any excess water from the bottom of the pan.

- Stir in the lemon juice and season to taste with salt and black pepper.

Makes 4 servings

Per serving: 79 calories, 4 g fat (1 g saturated), 9 g carbohydrates, 4 g fiber, 1 g sugars, 5 g protein

Crispy Oven-Baked Fries

You'll Need

2 medium russet potatoes
2 Tbsp. canola oil
Salt, to taste
2 cloves garlic, very finely minced
1 tsp. fresh rosemary leaves
¼ cup grated Parmesan

How to Make It

- Preheat the oven to 425°F.

- Peel the potatoes and cut into ¼-inch fries (about twice the thickness of standard fast-food fries). Soak in warm water for at least 15 minutes before cooking. Drain the potatoes and dry thoroughly.

- Combine the fries and the oil in a mixing bowl and toss until they're evenly coated. Season thoroughly with salt.

- Spread the fries out on a large baking sheet, being careful they don't overlap. Bake for 30 minutes, until the fries are just tender and lightly browned on the outside.

- Sprinkle with the garlic, rosemary, and Parmesan and return to the oven for another 10 minutes, until the cheese is melted and the garlic is lightly browned.

Makes 4 servings

Per serving: 150 calories, 9 g fat (0 g saturated), 15 g carbohydrates, 2 g fiber, 4 g sugars, 4 g protein

---

Turkey Chili

You'll Need

1 Tbsp. canola oil
1 large onion, chopped
2 cloves garlic, minced
1 tsp. ground cumin
½ tsp. dried oregano
¼ cup chili powder
⅛ tsp. ground cinnamon
2 bay leaves

2   lb. lean ground turkey
2   Tbsp. tomato paste
1   piece (about 1 oz.) dark chocolate or 1 Tbsp. cocoa powder
1   (12-oz.) bottle or can dark beer
1   Tbsp. chopped chipotle pepper
1   (28-oz.) can whole peeled tomatoes
1   (14-oz.) can white beans, rinsed and drained
1   (14-oz.) can pinto beans, rinsed and drained
Salt and black pepper, to taste
Hot sauce or cayenne (optional), to taste
Raw onions, shredded cheese, chopped scallions, lime wedges, sour
    cream (optional)

How to Make It

- Heat the oil in a large pot over medium heat. Add the onion and garlic and cook until the onion is translucent, about 5 minutes. Add the cumin, oregano, chili powder, cinnamon, and bay leaves and cook for another 2 to 3 minutes, until the spices are very fragrant.

- Add the turkey and tomato paste and stir with a wooden spoon until the turkey is no longer pink. Add the chocolate, beer, chipotle, and tomatoes, squeezing each tomato between your fingers so that it's chunky but not whole. Turn down the heat and simmer for 45 minutes.

- Add the beans and season with salt and pepper. Taste; if you like your chili hotter, add your favorite hot sauce or a few pinches of cayenne. Cook until the beans are hot. Serve topped with your choice of garnishes.

Makes 6 servings

Per serving: 324 calories, 5 g fat (1 g saturated), 34 g carbohydrates, 11 g fiber, 6 g sugars, 33 g protein

Herbed Roast Chicken with Root Vegetables

You'll Need

2   cloves garlic, minced
1   Tbsp. finely chopped fresh rosemary
Zest and juice of 1 lemon
1   Tbsp. olive oil, divided
1   chicken (4 lb.)
Salt and black pepper, to taste
1   large russet potato, sliced into ⅛-in. rounds
2   onions, quartered
4   large carrots, cut into large chunks

How to Make It

- Preheat the oven to 450°F. Mix the garlic, rosemary, lemon zest, and ½ tablespoon of the olive oil.

- Working on the chicken, gently separate the skin from the flesh at the bottom of the breast and spoon in half of the rosemary mixture; use your hands to spread it around as thoroughly as possible. Spread the remaining half over the top of the chicken and then season with plenty of salt and pepper.

- Mix the potato, onions, carrots, remaining olive oil, and a good pinch of salt and pepper. Arrange the vegetables in the bottom of a roasting pan and place the chicken on top, breast side up. Roast for 20 to 30 minutes, until the skin is lightly browned.

- Reduce the oven temperature to 350°F and roast for another 30 minutes or so. The chicken is done when the juices between the breast and the leg run clear and an instant-read thermometer inserted deep into the thigh reads 155°F.

- Remove from the oven and allow to rest for 10 minutes before carving. Serve with the vegetables.

Makes 4 servings

Per serving: 395 calories, 7.3 g fat (4.7 g saturated), 21 g carbohydrates, 4.5 g fiber, 26 g protein

Roast Pork Loin with Lemony White Beans

You'll Need

3   cloves garlic, minced

Zest of 2 oranges

1   Tbsp. fennel seeds

1½ Tbsp. chopped fresh rosemary, divided

1   Tbsp. olive oil

1   pork loin (2 lb.), preferably with a small rim of fat still attached

Salt and black pepper, to taste

2   (16-oz.) cans cannellini beans (aka great Northern or white kidney
     beans), rinsed and drained

Juice of 1 lemon

How to Make It

- Preheat the oven to 450°F. On a cutting board, combine the garlic,
  orange zest, fennel seeds, and 1 tablespoon of the rosemary. Run
  your knife repeatedly through the mix until it begins to take on a
  paste-like consistency. Scoop it up into a bowl and add the olive oil.
  Season the pork with salt and pepper, then rub it all over with the
  paste. At this point, you can cook it immediately or marinate the loin
  for up to 4 hours in the refrigerator for deeper flavor.

- Lay the pork in a roasting pan and roast for 25 to 30 minutes
  (depending on the thickness of the loin), until an instant-read
  thermometer inserted into the middle reads 150°F to 155°F. Remove
  from the oven and allow to rest for 10 minutes before slicing.

- While the pork rests, combine the beans, lemon juice, and the
  remaining ½ tablespoon of rosemary in a saucepan and cook until
  warm all the way through. Season with salt and pepper. Serve slices
  of the pork over the beans.

Makes 6 servings

Per serving: 323 calories, 8 g fat (2 g saturated), 23 g carbohydrates,
1 g fiber, 2 g sugars, 39 g protein

Pork Tenderloin with Grilled Pineapple Salsa

You'll Need

1 Tbsp. Dijon or grainy mustard
½ Tbsp. honey
½ Tbsp. chili powder
Salt and black pepper, to taste
1 lb. pork tenderloin
4½ -inch-thick slices pineapple, core removed
1 red onion, minced
1 jalapeño pepper, minced
½ cup chopped fresh cilantro
Juice of 1 lime

How to Make It

- Preheat the grill. Combine the mustard, honey, chili powder, salt, and pepper and rub all over the pork. Place the pork and pineapple slices on the grill. Grill the pineapple until lightly charred and softened. Grill the tenderloin, turning twice, for about 10 minutes. Let the pork rest for at least 5 minutes.

- Chop the pineapple into bite-size pieces. Combine with the onion, jalapeño, cilantro, and lime juice. Season with a bit of salt and pepper. Slice the pork and serve with the salsa.

Makes 4 servings

Per serving: 172 calories, 3 g fat (1 g saturated), 14 g carbohydrates, 2 g fiber, 10 g sugars, 23 g protein

Green Chile Cheeseburger

You'll Need

1 lb. ground sirloin or brisket
Salt and black pepper, to taste
1 can (4 oz) roasted green chiles, drained and chopped
4 slices Swiss cheese
4 large green leaf lettuce leaves
4 thick slices tomato
4 medium slices red onion

How to Make It

- Heat a grill, stovetop grill pan, or cast-iron skillet. Season the beef with salt and pepper. Form 4 patties, being careful not to overwork the meat.

- When the pan is hot, add the burgers. Cook for 3 to 4 minutes on the first side (until nicely charred), then flip and immediately. Top each with a tablespoon of chiles and a slice of Swiss. For medium-rare burgers, continue cooking for another 3 to 4 minutes, until the patties are just firm. Remove the burgers and allow to rest on a plate. Then place each burger in a large lettuce leaf and top with tomato and onion slices.

Makes 4 servings

Per serving: 316 calories, 19 g fat (9 g saturated), 5 g carbohydrates, 0 g fiber, 1 g sugars, 30 g protein

---

Seared Scallops with White Beans and Spinach

You'll Need
2 strips bacon
½ red onion, minced
1 clove garlic minced
1½ (14-oz.) cans white beans, rinsed and drained
4 cups baby spinach
1 lb. large sea scallops
Salt and black pepper, to taste
1 Tbsp. butter
Juice of 1 lemon

How to Make It

- Heat a medium saucepan over low heat. Cook the bacon until it has begun to crisp, then remove and chop into small pieces. Add the onion and garlic to the pan; sauté until the onion is soft and translucent, 2 to 3 minutes. Add the white beans and spinach and simmer until the beans are hot and the spinach is wilted. Keep warm.

- Heat a large cast-iron skillet or sauté pan over medium-high heat. Blot the scallops dry with a paper towel and season with salt and pepper on both sides. Add the butter and the scallops to the pan and sear the scallops for 2 to 3 minutes per side, until deeply caramelized.

- Before serving, add the lemon juice and bacon bits to the beans. Season with salt and pepper. Divide the beans among 4 warm bowls or plates and top with scallops.

Makes 4 servings

Per serving: 267 calories, 4 g fat (2 g saturated), 34 g carbohydrates, 9 g fiber, 2 g sugars, 27 g protein

---

Grilled Stuffed Portobello Mushrooms

You'll Need
4   portobello mushrooms, cleaned, stems removed
1   Tbsp. olive oil
2   Tbsp. balsamic vinegar
Salt and black pepper, to taste
2   medium tomatoes, chopped
¾   cup chopped fresh mozzarella
2   Tbsp. prepared pesto

How to Make It
- Preheat a grill over medium-low heat. Use a spoon to lightly scrape away some of the gills on the underside of the mushroom caps (this will create extra space for the filling). Place the mushrooms in a shallow baking dish, drizzle with the olive oil and balsamic vinegar, and season with salt and pepper. Combine the tomatoes, mozzarella, and pesto in a mixing bowl.

- Grill the portobellos, gill side down, for 2 minutes, then flip and fill each cap with the tomato mixture. Close the grill top and grill for another 8 to 10 minutes, until the mushrooms are soft and lightly charred and the mozzarella has melted.

Makes 4 servings

Per serving: 264 calories, 18 g fat (8 g saturated), 9 g carbohydrates, 2 g fiber, 4 g sugars, 14 g protein

11

The Belly Melt Fitness Plan

Boost your metabolism with our One Minute Morning Energizer and other simple exercises.

YOUR DIET AFFECTS your weight far more than your exercise routine ever will. So remember, don't expect exercise to cancel out those calories from your trip to the ice cream parlor. It won't. Sorry. While it's very easy to swallow 500 calories, it's very hard to burn off all those calories through exercise. (What makes it tougher is that the more you exercise, the hungrier you tend to become.)

More exercise is not the answer. But less exercise certainly can be. As we stressed earlier, you can only work out so much before you begin to hit a plateau; once you exceed 200 calories in energy expenditure, your body resets its metabolism to a slower burn as a protective measure to conserve energy and hamper weight loss. And store fat. So, too much exercise can work against you.

The secret to getting around this seemingly impossible barrier? Exercise *just enough*. The exercise plan in this chapter will make certain that you do the ideal amount of exercise to help you lose your belly rapidly while you also greatly improve your fitness level. Here's how it will happen: You will do a combination of brief workouts designed to burn fewer than 200 calories, including a full-body resistance-training workout that will put your high-protein diet to work building muscle and boosting your metabolism in ways that other exercise programs simply can't.

Every day of the week, you'll perform your One Minute Morning Energizer. Then, three times a week, you will do a 15- to 30-minute strength-training workout at home (or in a gym—your choice) using simple weights or exercise bands. On days when you don't strength train, you may want to walk, run, bike, or do some other optional interval-style cardio exercise for 10 to 30 minutes.

This may seem like a lot of exercise, but it's really not. The sessions are very short, however, they are *regular*, which is important for good health.

Don't panic: These workouts are short and simple, and so flexible that you can fit them in at any time of the day! They'll work with whatever energy level and time constraints you're dealing with.

Belly Melt Fitness Formula

Moving your body more every day + sticking to your meal plan will result in weight-loss success.

Here's a sample weekly schedule for getting there in 7 days:

EVERY DAY
One Minute Morning Energizer (even on rest day)

DAY 1
Tone & Strengthen Workout (15 to 30 minutes)

DAY 2
Interval Cardio Workout (10 to 30 minutes)

DAY 3
Tone & Strengthen Workout

DAY 4
Interval Cardio Workout

DAY 5
Tone & Strengthen Workout

DAY 6
Interval Cardio Workout

DAY 7
Rest

One Minute Morning Energizer

This is your no-excuses opportunity to reap the benefits of exercise without spending a lot of time going to the gym. It works for everyone and it's ideal for people who are overweight or don't exercise regularly because it involves just one minute of intense exercise broken into 20-second spurts over a 6-minute period of activity.

It's based on studies at McMaster University in Ontario. Researchers there knew that brief bouts of intense exercise interspersed with much slower recovery segments provide a great metabolic lift to burn calories as well as improve measures of endurance and cardiovascular health. What they wanted to find out was the minimum amount of effort you could exert to reap the fitness benefits of much longer exercise sessions. They decided that 30 seconds of all-out effort was just too long for many overweight and out-of-shape people to sustain so they tried cutting that intense segment by a third, and sure enough, it worked.

What this means for you: Three 20-second bouts of all-out physical effort (or you might call it one cumulative minute of hell), in between slow, easy bouts of recovery movement are all you need to gain significant physical benefits of exercise. So we developed the One Minute Morning Energizer quickie workout for you to do every morning before your smoothie breakfast. It's superfast and it will get you in the groove to move more throughout the day and even try the additional workouts you'll find later in this chapter. Use your smartphone's stopwatch function or the second hand of a clock to keep track of your time as you do your Morning Energizer. Here are a couple of ways to get it done:

Morning Energizer Option #1:
Walking, running or cycling, or exercising on a stationary bike, treadmill, or other cardio machine...

- Warm-up (2 minutes)—Walk or pedal at an easy pace or do one minute of marching in place and one of jumping jacks.

- High-intensity interval (20 seconds)—Exercise at a high intensity. Pedal, walk, or run as fast and hard as you can while maintaining control and good form. We're talking about all-out effort. Don't hold anything back for a full 20 seconds. At the end, you should be huffing and puffing to catch your breath.

- Recovery (60 seconds)—Exercise at a recovery pace. Slow way down to a very easy pace. Don't stop; keep pedaling or walking slowly until your breathing returns to a normal, comfortable rate. As you near the 90-second mark, start to ramp up your intensity again.

- High-intensity interval (20 seconds)—Exercise at a high intensity.

- Recovery (60 seconds)—Exercise at a recovery pace.

- High-intensity interval (20 seconds)—Exercise at a high intensity.

- Recovery (60 seconds). You're done!

Morning Energizer Option #2:
In a small room, using only your body weight...

- Warm-up (2 minutes)—Warm up by marching in place. Swing your arms and lift your knees so your thighs rise to nearly parallel with the floor. Do this at an easy pace for one minute then switch to jumping jacks for one minute.

- High-intensity interval (20 seconds)—Exercise at a high intensity. Choose one of the body-weight exercises starting on page 142 and do it as fast and hard as you can while maintaining control and good form. We're talking about all-out effort. Don't hold anything back for a full 20 seconds. At the end, you should be huffing and puffing to catch your breath.

- Recovery (60 seconds)—March in place slowly until your breathing returns to normal.

- High-intensity interval (20 seconds)—Exercise at a high intensity using the exercise of your choice.

- Recovery (60 seconds)—March in place slowly until your breathing returns to normal.
- High-intensity interval (20 seconds)—Exercise at a high intensity using the exercise of your choice.
- Recovery (60 seconds). You're done!

If you've chosen Energizer Option #2, select from these body-weight exercises to complete the 20-second high-intensity interval portions of your One Minute Morning Energizer.

Body-Weight Exercises

Arms-Up Squat
- Spread your feet shoulder-width apart with toes pointed slightly outward. Raise both arms above your head. Keeping arms raised, bend your knees and push your butt back as if sitting in a chair. Lower your body until your thighs are parallel with the floor. Pause a second and quickly straighten your legs to stand. Repeat immediately and quickly for 20 seconds.

Superhero Squat Jump
- Do the Arms-Up Squat as described above, except from the squat position, explosively press your feet into the floor to jump as high as you can (or as high as your ceiling will allow). When your feet hit the ground, go immediately into the next squat. Repeat squat jumps as fast as possible for 20 seconds.

Seal Jack
- This variation of the jumping jack is good for those who experience pain when raising arms overhead during the traditional exercise. (Use it as part of your warm-up or as an intense exercise. Start by standing with feet together and placing your palms on your chest with elbows spread and arms

parallel to the floor. As you jump to spread your legs outward, simultaneously swing your arms out to the sides so they are parallel with the floor. Jump your feet back while swinging your arms back to your chest. Do these as quickly as you can for 20 seconds.

Push-Up

- This classic chest/arms/abs exercise will elevate your heart rate very quickly if done fast. Get into a plank position, with your arms straight, hands on the floor directly underneath your shoulders, and your toes on the floor behind you. Your body should be arrow-straight from your heels to your head. Without dipping or lifting your butt, lower yourself until your chest nearly touches the floor and then immediately press yourself back to the starting position. Repeat for 20 seconds. These are tough. To make them easier, you can do modified push-ups by kneeling or hands-elevated push-up by placing your hands on the edge of a bathtub or chair, which will reduce the amount of weight you'll be pushing. To make push-ups more metabolic, push off the floor explosively so that your hands come off the floor. For an even greater challenge, throw in a clap before your hands return to the floor.

Reverse Lunge

- Stand straight with feet hip-width apart, hands on your hips. Take a big step backward with your right leg and press the ball of your right foot to the floor as you slowly lower your body by bending your left leg. Lower until your left leg forms a right angle and your right knee hovers an inch above the floor. Next, press back into a standing position and bring your right foot forward. Repeat the move by stepping back with your left foot. Continue alternating this way for 20 seconds. To make this exercise more challenging, hold a dumbbell in each hand. Don't have weights? Hold a gallon jug of water in each hand as you do the exercise.

Mountain Climber

- Get into the "up" push-up position with your hands directly under your shoulders and arms straight. Now rapidly bend and straighten each leg one at a time in alternating fashion. It's like running in place with your hands on the ground. Try bringing your knees to your chest with each pump of your legs. Do these as fast as possible for a full 20 seconds.

Burpee

- This advanced exercise is similar to the squat thrust you performed in high school gym class. And it's a great way to crank up the intensity. Stand with feet hip-width apart. Bend at the knees and waist to place your hands shoulder-width apart on the floor in front of you. Quickly jump your feet back so you end up in a plank position. (Optional step: Do a push-up at this point.) Then jump your feet back under you and straighten your legs to jump back to a standing position. Repeat rapidly for 20 seconds.

Do your One Minute Morning Energizer every morning—even on weekends. If you are out of shape, this simple six-minute session (one minute hard/five minutes easy) will help you build up your cardiovascular fitness very quickly. And you'll find a funny thing happening: You'll like the feeling and want to do more!

Tone & Strengthen Workout

Strength training builds stronger muscles. The type of strength-training workout in this plan *will not* give you the hulky-bulky muscles that make you look like a comic-book superhero. By building stronger muscle mass in this plan, you'll make your body look firmer, tighter, more toned, and healthier. Just what you want! And because muscle mass burns more calories than fat (not a lot, but every little bit counts!), the more muscle on your skeleton, the quicker you will lose the fat throughout your body, especially abdominal fat.

Strength training is doubly important as we age. With each passing decade, your body naturally loses muscle mass and, if you're not careful about reducing your calorie consumption accordingly, replaces it with fat. Strength training and strong muscles offer many other health and weight-loss benefits: They boost your energy level, making everyday tasks easier. Strong muscle helps your body react quickly in emergency situations, such as when you trip over a curb and need to step quickly to catch your balance before you do a face-plant on the sidewalk. Strength training also triggers your body to grow stronger, denser bones, which combats the bone loss that accelerates especially in women as they age. Muscle helps your body metabolize blood sugar, as well, reducing your risk of developing type 2 diabetes. Strength training improves sleep quality, too.

Are you convinced that strength training is something you absolutely *must* do, not only to lose your belly rapidly, but also to bulletproof your body as you get older? We are. That's why we developed this easy resistance workout especially for people who may not be familiar with traditional weight-training exercises. You can do it at home or at the gym. This is a resistance workout, meaning you will stress your muscles against resistance by holding light dumbbells, gallon water jugs, or by using exercise bands.

Stressing a muscle against resistance causes tiny pain-free micro-tears in muscle tissue. At night while you're asleep, your body will repair those microscopic injuries. It's a process that builds and strengthens muscle.

To do this workout at home, if you don't already own them, you'll need to purchase dumbbells and elastic fitness bands from a sporting goods supplier. Dumbbells come in many different weights—a pair of 8- to 10-pound dumbbells will be fine for these exercises. Dumbbells hold one distinct advantage over their barbell cousins. Because your hands aren't fixed in relation to one other, as with a barbell, with dumbbells you can work each side of your body independently of the other.

The freedom of motion that dumbbells allow helps you to work around any joint injuries or flexibility issues you may have. Plus, they help you develop both symmetry and stability. The exercise descriptions below are for dumbbells or water-filled gallon jugs. You can easily adapt them for use with resistance bands.

Tone & Strengthen Step-by-Step

For a simple total-body strength workout, always begin with a 3-minute warm-up of either stationary cycling or body-weight calisthenics like jumping jacks and skater hops. Next, do 3 sets (unless noted) of 8 to 12 repetitions of each of the following exercises. Rest for about 30 seconds between exercises. Complete all 3 sets of one exercise before moving on to the next.

1) WARM UP
Jumping Jack

* Stand straight with your feet hip-width apart and hands at your sides. Simultaneously raise your arms above your head as you jump and spread your feet shoulder-width apart. Jump your feet back to center while lowering arms to your sides. Repeat quickly.

Skater Hop

* Start with your feet together. Push off with your left foot to hop laterally to the right about 3 feet. Land on your right foot and follow by swinging your left behind you. Immediately hop back, pushing off your right foot, landing on your left and trailing your right foot behind you. Swing your arms with each hop in an ice-skating motion.

2) TOTAL-BODY STRENGTH MOVES
Plank or Push-Up

* 1 set for Plank; 3 sets, 8–10 reps for Push-Up (or Step Push-Up)

Plank

* Get on all fours and then extend your legs out straight behind you. Your hands should be directly under your shoulders. Straighten your arms. Brace your core and keep your back flat, forming a straight line from your heels to your head. Hold this rigid position for 30 to 60 seconds.

Push-Up

* Get into a plank position with your palms on the floor directly under your shoulders and your arms straight. Your back should be flat and rigid from your heels to your head. Brace your core. This will help you maintain proper form and burn more calories because you are engaging more muscle fibers. Bend your arms to lower yourself toward the floor until your chest is about an inch from the floor. Press yourself up explosively. Repeat.

Step Push-Up Get into a push-up position, but instead of placing your hands on the floor, place them on a stair-step, bench, or other stable structure that's raised off the floor. Keep your back arrow-straight from heels to head. Your arms should be extended straight. Brace your abs. Bend your elbows to lower yourself until your chest is an inch off the step. Pause a second, then push yourself up. Repeat.

Dumbbell Squat
3 sets, 8–10 reps

- Hold a 10-pound dumbbell in each hand at your sides, palms facing in. Stand with your feet spread shoulder-width apart with toes pointed slightly outward. Bend your knees and push your butt back as if trying to close a door behind you. Lower your body until your thighs are parallel with the floor. Pause a second, then quickly straighten your legs to stand. Repeat.

Flutter Kick
3 sets, 10 reps

- Lie on your back on the floor with your arms straight, palms down next to your sides, and toes pointed. Engage your abs to lift your feet about a foot off the floor. Keeping your legs rigid, begin quickly flutter kicking your straight legs back and forth as you would while swimming. Four kicks equals one rep. Repeat.

Dumbbell Biceps Curl
3 sets, 8–10 reps

- Stand with your feet hip-width apart and hold a 5- to 10-pound dumbbell in each hand at your sides, palms facing in. Simultaneously bend both arms to raise the dumbbells to your shoulders. As you slowly raise the weights, rotate your hands so your thumbs face away from your body by the time the weights reach the front of your shoulders. Note: Your upper arms should remain stationary against your body throughout the movement. Pause, then slowly lower the weights while rotating your hands inward so that your palms face the sides of your thighs by the time your arms are straight. Repeat.

Dumbbell Forward Lunge
3 sets, 8-10 reps

- Stand with your feet together and hold a dumbbell in each hand at your sides, palms facing in. Take a large step forward with your right leg and lower your body toward the floor. Your front leg should bend at the knee forming a right angle. Your back leg should be bent slightly. Lower yourself until your back knee hovers an inch above the ground and your right thigh is parallel with the floor. Pause in this position for a second. Press your right foot into the floor to push yourself back to the starting position. Next, step forward with your left foot and repeat.

Dumbbell Push Press
3 sets, 8-10 reps

- Stand with your feet shoulder-width apart and hold a dumbbell in each hand at your shoulders, elbows bent, palms facing in. Bend your knees to dip down slightly into a half squat. Press your feet into the floor to aggressively stand while straightening your arms overhead. (Straightening your legs will provide momentum to help you press the weights overhead.) Slowly lower the weights to your shoulders and repeat.

Side Plank (right side)
1 set, 30- to 60-second hold

- Lie on the floor on your right side, stacking your left leg over your right and propping yourself up on your right elbow and forearm. Your elbow should be directly under your shoulder. Place your left hand on your hip. Brace your core and lift your hips off the floor so that your body forms a rigid straight line. Don't allow your hips to sag. Hold this position for 30 to 60 seconds, then release to the floor.

Dumbbell Standing Triceps Press
3 sets, 8–10 reps

- Stand with feet shoulder-width apart and hold a dumbbell in each hand. Press the dumbbells above your head so your arms are straight and palms are facing in. Keeping your upper arms against your ears, move only your forearms by bending at the elbows to lower the weights simultaneously behind your head. Once your forearms meet your biceps, press the weights back up until your arms are straight again, being careful to move only your forearms. Repeat.

Side Plank (left side)
1 set, 30- to 60-second hold

- Lie on the floor on your left side, stacking your right leg over your left and propping yourself up on your left elbow and forearm. Your elbow should be directly under your shoulder. Place your right hand on your hip. Brace your core and lift your hips off the floor so that your body forms a rigid straight line. Don't allow your hips to sag. Hold this position for 30 to 60 seconds, then release to the floor.

Optional Cardio Workouts

For another great way to boost your fat-burning metabolism and improve your health without sacrificing muscle, give one or more of these optional cardio workouts a try. They use the same high-intensity interval-training concept you employ with your One Minute Morning Energizer session. You alternate short bursts of faster, high-intensity activity with bouts of slower, lower-intensity "recovery" periods. Many scientific studies have shown that this type of exercise is highly effective for weight loss and for targeting belly fat. Consider this Danish study reported by the American Diabetes Association: Two groups of people with type 2 diabetes were put on a walking program. One group walked at a steady speed, while the other group varied its walking speeds. After four months, the interval-training group lost eight more pounds than the steady-pace walkers. Even better, the walkers who changed up their speeds lost visceral belly fat and improved their blood sugar control.

Here are two simple walking intervals you can do just about anywhere and a third to do on sturdy bleachers or on longer sets of stairs...

1) 10-Minute Walking Interval

- Warm up (2 minutes)—Warm up by walking at a slow, easy pace.
- Move all-out (30 seconds)—Walk fast, pumping your arms to engage your entire body.
- Recover (60 seconds)—Slow down to a moderate pace to lower your heart rate.

- Move all-out (60 seconds)—Walk fast.

- Recover (2 minutes)—Slow to a moderate pace.
  You should be able to talk in complete sentences.

- Move all-out (30 seconds)—Walk fast.

- Cool down (3 minutes)—Slow to a moderate pace.

2) 30-Minute Walking Interval

- Warm up (3 minutes)—Warm up by walking at a slow pace.

- Move all-out (60 seconds)—Walk fast.

- Recover (2 minutes)—Slow to a moderate pace maintained with easy effort.

- Move all-out (60 seconds)—Walk fast.

- Recover (2 minutes)—Slow to a moderate pace maintained with easy effort.

- Move all-out (60 seconds)—Walk fast.

- Recover (2 minutes)—Slow to a moderate pace maintained with easy effort.

- Move all-out (60 seconds)—Walk fast.

- Recover (2 minutes)—Slow to a moderate pace maintained with easy effort.

- Move all-out (60 seconds)—Walk fast.

- Recover (2 minutes)—Slow to a moderate pace maintained with easy effort.

- Move all-out (60 seconds)—Walk fast.

- Recover (2 minutes)—Slow to a moderate pace maintained with easy effort.

- Move all-out (60 seconds)—Walk fast.

- Recover (2 minutes)—Slow to a moderate pace maintained with easy effort.

- Move all-out (60 seconds)—Walk fast.
- Recover (60 seconds)—Slow to a moderate pace maintained with easy effort.
- Move all-out (60 seconds)—Walk fast.
- Cool down (3 minutes)—Slow to cooldown pace.

3) 10-Minute Stair-Climbing Interval

- Another way to increase the metabolic intensity of a walking workout and shorten workout time is to make walking harder. Do that with a stair-climbing interval workout. Use the stadium bleachers of a local athletic field or the stairs at your workplace. You don't go very fast. Climbing the stairs will force a high-intensity effort. Staircases have roughly a 65-percent grade, which will force you to exert much more leg strength to lift your body weight. Warm up by walking on flat ground at a slow pace for two minutes. Walk up the stairs (at least 10 stairs) quickly but in control. Walk down at a moderate pace and repeat. To progress, try taking every other stair step going up. It's an explosive movement that generates a lot of leg power.

12

What's Next?

Follow these final bits of advice to maintain your body beyond the 7-Day Belly Melt Diet.

BY THE TIME your seven days of structured eating and exercise are complete, you should be able to measure a significant change in your body weight and the size of your belly. (If you aren't where you'd like to be, we recommend reviewing your food/water/fitness log, looking for areas that need improvement, and following the 7-day program once more.)

One of the reasons the 7-Day Belly Melt Diet works so well to help you lose belly fat quickly is that it's a strategic, step-by-step system that's easy to follow for a brief period. By following the meal plan and rules for slashing calories, you are forced to become very mindful of your eating and fitness behaviors. You have a top-of-mind goal (to fit into those jeans) and a deadline looming (that high school reunion or other highly motivating social event) and an easy-to-follow-daily structure. In short, you are ultra-aware of this exciting new way of living. But what happens after the reunion or beach vacation is over? Do you go back to unhealthy eating habits?

This seven-day plan isn't like cramming for a final exam in calculus, something you may never use again. On the contrary, you want to eat smarter and healthier for life. So we designed the Belly Melt Diet to be something you use to set a short-term goal that you can build upon and, more importantly, sustain for the rest of your life. Sure, you may not want to have a smoothie for breakfast every day from now to eternity. Your body will crave a big breakfast of bacon and eggs, home fries, and maybe even a blueberry pancake now and then, especially on a chilly Sunday morning. Remember, this isn't about sacrificial dieting. Success comes from mindful eating. After seven days on the plan, you should have gotten into an easy, effortless rhythm of habits that just feel right. Let's review what you've accomplished:

- You've established the habit of moving your body more every day.

- You've recognized the power of protein (through your morning smoothie) to satisfy your hunger and ward off cravings.

- You've learned how to avoid extreme hunger (which can trigger bingeing) by eating every three or four hours (six feedings).

- You've realized how little water you've been drinking and changed that shortfall by really making an effort to down 16 glasses of water daily.

- If you drink, you may have realized how much alcohol you had been drinking, and you've learned that cutting out the wine, beer, and cocktails is the easiest way to lose weight superfast.

- You've switched from sweetened beverages to unsweetened drinks such as flavonoid-rich iced tea.

- You've learned how to use your dinner plate as a visual template of what to eat and how much.

- You've become aware of the importance of eating more flavonoid-rich F.L.A.V.O.R. foods to harness their ability to reduce inflammation in your arteries and turn off the genes that cause fat storage.

- You've discovered the time-saving secret of interval training for cardiovascular health and the fat-burning power of building muscle through strength training.

- You've become much more mindful of the food choices you make every day and how critical they are to staying lean.

In short, you've accomplished a heck of a lot in seven days. And the good news is that those established habits should be easy to sustain because they are easy to remember and they automatically reduce the cravings that often encourages overeating.

But let's say despite your successes you start to drift in

the other direction. You'll know without even stepping on a scale because your clothes will start to feel a little tighter. That's a sign that you simply need to embark on another short 7-day cycle of the program. (Don't forget to take a new photo of yourself and sign a contract promise just as you did in the beginning; it'll help!) And remind yourself that success means more than reaching a goal weight or dress size. Success means better health, more energy to enjoy life, and feeling happy and confident in your body. That's what eating whole or minimally processed foods and lean proteins will do for you automatically if you continue to strengthen your habit of mindful eating.

Let's review the rules that will guide you to stay on track for life:

A Sensible Plan for Life

Rule #1: Fill your lunch and dinner plates using the pie chart method, aka the 25/75 guideline, most of the time.

Anytime you want to lose weight, you have to reduce the number of calories you consume. But calorie counting is unpleasant. To do it effectively, you need to know two things: the recommended serving size and the number of calories in a serving. Unless you like measuring and weighing your food, it's a real hassle and not the way to enjoy food. That's why, as important as calorie reduction is for rapid weight loss, we encourage you to avoid counting calories. Instead, we devised two tricks to help guarantee that you automatically select the right amounts of protein and low-calorie, high-fiber carbohydrates. Rule #1 employs the first trick—the pie chart plate guideline, which should be very familiar to you by now.

To review, this is a simple way to eyeball proper portion size. For lunch and dinner visually divide your plate into one-quarter lean protein (meat, poultry, fish, pork or legumes like lentils or chickpeas) and three-quarters vegetables and fruits. That's it. Filling your plate that way automatically ensures that you are fueling your body with hunger-satisfying, muscle-building protein and you're loading up on fiber- and nutrient-rich vegetables and fruits. And without making a big deal of it, you end up eliminating the temptation of highly processed starches, which typically boost blood sugar and trigger cravings. The 25/75 plate guideline is an easy trick for glancing at any meal and determining if it fits your diet.

The second trick for filling your belly is employing the acronym we learned at the beginning of the 7-Day Belly Melt Diet: F.L.A.V.O.R., which stands for:

- **F** reshly Brewed Tea
- **L** entils and Beans
- **A** pples, Berries, and Other Fruits
- **V** egetables and Leafy Greens
- **O** ils, Nuts, and Seeds
- **R** ed meat and Other Protein Sources

Focus on these foods anytime you fill up your plate and you will automatically fill your belly with hunger-satisfying foods packed with nutrition, specifically those powerfully healthful compounds called flavonoids that we talked about in Chapter 3.

Rule #2: Eat something every three to four hours.

Some people graze all day long. That's not a bad thing if what they're munching on is mostly kale and celery, but when it's chips, hunks of cheese, coffee cake, and milk chocolate, calories add up and blood sugar levels rise. Our plan calls for three meals and three snacks a day. When you eat that often, you naturally space your feeding times to three, maybe four, hours apart—roughly the time it takes for you to digest what you ate and start getting hungry again.

The goal is to keep your belly satisfied (protein and fiber will do that) to avoid cravings and eating binges. Your busy day might force you to miss a meal or snack now and then. Don't worry about it, but take notice of how your body reacts when that happens. Are you craving sugary baked goods or fatty snacks? Make a note in your journal. That's part of becoming a more mindful eater. Be aware of what causes hunger and which foods and meal schedules maintain the status quo.

Rule #3: Avoid drinks with calories most of the time.

Following this single rule is one of the most effective ways to reduce your calorie consumption and lose both weight and belly fat. It may help for you to know this alarming fact: Sugary drinks are the single-largest source of calories in the American diet. Keep this visual in mind when faced with a choice of, say, a sugary soft drink or a glass of unsweetened iced tea: A 12-ounce can of soda contains nine teaspoons of added sugars, while the more popular 20-ounce bottle contains 16 teaspoons. And choosing diet soda or sugar-free fruit-flavored drinks doesn't help. One recent study from Johns Hopkins found that people who drink diet beverages end up consuming more calories from food than people who drink regular soda or other sugary beverages. Why? The body expects calories when it tastes something sweet, and when it doesn't get the calories from that tricky artificial sweetener, it craves calories from another source, encouraging you to eat more.

On the Belly Melt Diet, we want you to drink lots of unsweetened tea for the powerful fat-fighting nutrients in tea and up to a gallon of ice water a day. Why? First, remember that thirst is often confused with hunger. If you're craving a doughnut, it may be that you're simply dehydrated. Try drinking a glass of ice water and waiting a few minutes. Are you still hungry now? When you're hydrated, chances are good that those false hunger pangs will be gone. If they aren't, then go have a snack.

Beer, wine, and margaritas are also loaded with calories, and the alcohol in those beverages encourages fat storage. That's why we encouraged you to avoid alcohol during the 7-Day Belly Melt Diet. Doing so cuts calorie consumption dramatically if you regularly imbibe. But if you can't see yourself going through life without a glass of wine with dinner or a cocktail with friends, we're not going to be party poopers. After you've reached your goal weight, you can reintroduce adult beverages. Just keep in mind that as we mentioned before, the more alcohol you drink, the harder it will be to maintain a flat belly and stay at your goal weight.

Rule #4: Maintain muscle, and exercise for health, not for weight loss.
Hopefully, we've convinced you to pick up the weights and do some regular resistance training. After age 30, your body naturally loses about one to two percent of its muscle per decade. That is, unless you do something about it. Building

muscle is important for a number of reasons: When you lose muscle due to lack of use or what's known as sarcopenia, age-related muscle loss, the empty space left behind is often replaced by fat. Even if you are relatively thin, if you lose the muscle you have, you can become *skinny fat*, which is unhealthy.

Muscle, as we've learned, is more metabolically active than fat, so the more you have on your frame, the more calories you burn even at rest. Besides, a strong, muscular body is a body more likely to be in motion, and movement is a key component of good cardiovascular health. So try to do resistance training with body weight or actual weight-lifting equipment two or three times a week.

Ideally, you are still doing your One Minute Morning Energizer routine, described in Chapter 11. It's a great way to wake up and jump-start your metabolism for the day, and it exposes you to the time-saving, endurance-strengthening benefits of high-intensity interval training. To maintain a healthy body as you age, get in the habit of doing a brief interval session every day. You can do it through walking, running, biking, stair climbing, weight lifting, or just about any physical activity that allows you to quickly speed up to heart-pounding effort and slow down to a resting pace.

Okay, so you've got it? That's the simple plan to maintain that flat belly and the healthy, exuberantly energetic body you've built while on the 7-Day Belly Melt Diet. It's simple enough to maintain for life and easy enough to intensify should you ever again need to flatten your belly and lose a few pounds ARAP—as rapidly as possible. The object is to stay lean and healthy so you can enjoy life for as long as possible.

A

The 7-Day Belly Melt Diet Food & Fitness Tracker

IF YOU'VE PLAYED golf, you know it's a complicated game to master. Scoring golf, however, is pretty simple. On a scorecard, you mark the final number of hits per hole for each player. At the end of 18 holes, the lowest score wins.

It's simple. So, you might wonder, why bother with the card? Can't everyone just keep count of their own hits?

Well, if you know any golfers, you know they're a competitive bunch, and some have been known to cheat by "forgetting" to record a stroke now and then. So the scorecard keeps everyone accountable. But there's more to it than just keeping an accurate score. The scorecard is also very useful for improving one's game.

A smart duffer will keep track of how many short approach shots and putts he needed on each hole to point out flaws in his short game. Some golfers will draw the shape of each drive and at the end of the day count how many went left, middle, right, or right into the woods. Scribbles, statistics, and notes on a scorecard help a golfer recognize habits and fix mistakes as well as provide motivation to practice.

This food and fitness tracker will do the same sort of thing for you. Taking the time to track your progress can make a difference. It's an accountability tool. Studies have proven that people who log the foods they consume and keep track of their weight are more successful than people who do not. In one study at the University of Arkansas, dieters who kept a food record for three weeks lost three-and-one-half pounds more than those who didn't.

One of the greatest benefits to keeping track of your food is that it forces you to become hyperaware of what you are putting in your mouth. That cupcake or margarita is right there in black and white for you to see and remember. And you can attach a calorie number to it. In short order, you become a more mindful eater. You grow to recognize how certain foods impact your body. What's more, tracking weight and waist measurements provides regular positive feedback, which is powerful motivation.

To be successful in your weight-loss journey, you need to have a goal weight or body shape you want to achieve and you need a starting reference point. So, for starters, grab a tape measure and find a scale. Fill out the following chart so that you have something accurate to compare it to seven days from now, and again, say in six months.

YOUR STARTING MEASUREMENTS

DATE:_____

TIME OF DAY: _____

HEIGHT: _____

WEIGHT:_____

WAIST (Circumference in inches at belly button):

_____

HIPS (Circumference in inches at widest part of hips):

_____

WAIST-TO-HIP RATIO:_____

LEFT THIGH: _____

RIGHT THIGH:_____

The 7-Day Lose Your Belly Diet Food & Fitness Tracker

DAY 1

DATE:_____

BREAKFAST:

_____

_____

Rate your hunger before:
1 2 3 4 5 6 7 8 9 10 (10 = famished)

Rate your hunger after:
1 2 3 4 5 6 7 8 9 10 (1 = totally satisfied)

SNACK #1:

_____

_____

Rate your hunger before:
1 2 3 4 5 6 7 8 9 10 (10 = famished)

Rate your hunger after:
1 2 3 4 5 6 7 8 9 10 (1 = totally satisfied)

LUNCH:

_____

_____

Rate your hunger before:

1 2 3 4 5 6 7 8 9 10 (10 = famished)

Rate your hunger after:

1 2 3 4 5 6 7 8 9 10 (1 = totally satisfied)

SNACK #2:

_____

_____

Rate your hunger before:

1 2 3 4 5 6 7 8 9 10 (10 = famished)

Rate your hunger after:

1 2 3 4 5 6 7 8 9 10 (1 = totally satisfied)

DESSERT OR SNACK #3:
TIME EATEN:

_____

_____

DAILY WATER (check boxes; aim for sixteen 8-oz glasses):

☐ ☐ ☐ ☐ ☐ ☐ ☐ ☐ ☐ ☐ ☐ ☐ ☐ ☐ ☐ ☐

EXERCISE
DATE: _____

MORNING ENERGIZER:

Check option A ☐ , or option B ☐

Strength Training (list exercises):
repetitions / sets

_____

_____ / _____

_____

_____ / _____

_____

_____ / _____

_____

_____ / _____

_____

_____ / _____

OPTIONAL CARDIO INTERVAL
OR OTHER PHYSICAL ACTIVITY:

_____

_____ / _____

_____

_____ / _____

DAY 2

DATE:_____

BREAKFAST:

_____

_____

Rate your hunger before:
1 2 3 4 5 6 7 8 9 10 (10 = famished)

Rate your hunger after:
1 2 3 4 5 6 7 8 9 10 (1 = totally satisfied)

SNACK #1:

_____

_____

Rate your hunger before:
1 2 3 4 5 6 7 8 9 10 (10 = famished)

Rate your hunger after:
1 2 3 4 5 6 7 8 9 10 (1 = totally satisfied)

LUNCH:

_____

_____

Rate your hunger before:
1 2 3 4 5 6 7 8 9 10 (10 = famished)

Rate your hunger after:
1 2 3 4 5 6 7 8 9 10 (1 = totally satisfied)

SNACK #2:

_____

_____

Rate your hunger before:
1 2 3 4 5 6 7 8 9 10 (10 = famished)
Rate your hunger after:
1 2 3 4 5 6 7 8 9 10 (1 = totally satisfied)

DESSERT OR SNACK #3:
TIME EATEN:

_____

_____

DAILY WATER (check boxes; aim for sixteen 8-oz glasses):

☐ ☐ ☐ ☐ ☐ ☐ ☐ ☐ ☐ ☐ ☐ ☐ ☐ ☐ ☐ ☐

EXERCISE
DATE: _____

MORNING ENERGIZER:

Check option A ☐ , or option B ☐

Strength Training (list exercises):
repetitions / sets

_____

_____ / _____

_____

_____ / _____

_____

_____ / _____

_____

_____ / _____

_____

_____ / _____

OPTIONAL CARDIO INTERVAL
OR OTHER PHYSICAL ACTIVITY:

_____

_____ / _____

_____

_____ / _____

DAY 3

DATE:_____

BREAKFAST:

_____

_____

Rate your hunger before:
1 2 3 4 5 6 7 8 9 10 (10 = famished)
Rate your hunger after:
1 2 3 4 5 6 7 8 9 10 (1 = totally satisfied)

SNACK #1:

_____

_____

Rate your hunger before:
1 2 3 4 5 6 7 8 9 10 (10 = famished)
Rate your hunger after:
1 2 3 4 5 6 7 8 9 10 (1 = totally satisfied)

LUNCH:

_____

_____

Rate your hunger before:
1 2 3 4 5 6 7 8 9 10 (10 = famished)
Rate your hunger after:
1 2 3 4 5 6 7 8 9 10 (1 = totally satisfied)

SNACK #2:

_____

_____

Rate your hunger before:
1 2 3 4 5 6 7 8 9 10 (10 = famished)
Rate your hunger after:
1 2 3 4 5 6 7 8 9 10 (1 = totally satisfied)

DESSERT OR SNACK #3:
TIME EATEN:

_____

_____

DAILY WATER (check boxes; aim for sixteen 8-oz glasses):

☐ ☐ ☐ ☐ ☐ ☐ ☐ ☐ ☐ ☐ ☐ ☐ ☐ ☐ ☐ ☐

EXERCISE
DATE: _____

MORNING ENERGIZER:

Check option A ☐ , or option B ☐

Strength Training (list exercises):
repetitions / sets

_____

_____ / _____

_____

_____ / _____

_____

_____ / _____

_____

_____ / _____

_____

_____ / _____

OPTIONAL CARDIO INTERVAL
OR OTHER PHYSICAL ACTIVITY:

_____

_____ / _____

_____

_____ / _____

DAY 4

DATE: _____

BREAKFAST:

_____

_____

Rate your hunger before:
1 2 3 4 5 6 7 8 9 10 (10 = famished)
Rate your hunger after:
1 2 3 4 5 6 7 8 9 10 (1 = totally satisfied)

SNACK #1:

_____

_____

Rate your hunger before:
1 2 3 4 5 6 7 8 9 10 (10 = famished)
Rate your hunger after:
1 2 3 4 5 6 7 8 9 10 (1 = totally satisfied)

LUNCH:

_____

_____

Rate your hunger before:
1 2 3 4 5 6 7 8 9 10 (10 = famished)
Rate your hunger after:
1 2 3 4 5 6 7 8 9 10 (1 = totally satisfied)

SNACK #2:

_____

_____

Rate your hunger before:
1 2 3 4 5 6 7 8 9 10 (10 = famished)
Rate your hunger after:
1 2 3 4 5 6 7 8 9 10 (1 = totally satisfied)

DESSERT OR SNACK #3:
TIME EATEN:

_____

_____

DAILY WATER (check boxes; aim for sixteen 8-oz glasses):

☐ ☐ ☐ ☐ ☐ ☐ ☐ ☐ ☐ ☐ ☐ ☐ ☐ ☐ ☐ ☐

EXERCISE
DATE: _____

MORNING ENERGIZER:

Check option A ☐ , or option B ☐

Strength Training (list exercises):
repetitions / sets

_____

_____ / _____

_____

_____ / _____

_____

_____ / _____

_____

_____ / _____

_____

_____ / _____

OPTIONAL CARDIO INTERVAL
OR OTHER PHYSICAL ACTIVITY:

_____

_____ / _____

_____

_____ / _____

DAY 5

DATE:_____

BREAKFAST:

_____

_____

Rate your hunger before:
1 2 3 4 5 6 7 8 9 10 (10 = famished)
Rate your hunger after:
1 2 3 4 5 6 7 8 9 10 (1 = totally satisfied)

SNACK #1:

_____

_____

Rate your hunger before:
1 2 3 4 5 6 7 8 9 10 (10 = famished)
Rate your hunger after:
1 2 3 4 5 6 7 8 9 10 (1 = totally satisfied)

LUNCH:

_____

_____

Rate your hunger before:
1 2 3 4 5 6 7 8 9 10 (10 = famished)
Rate your hunger after:
1 2 3 4 5 6 7 8 9 10 (1 = totally satisfied)

SNACK #2:

_____

_____

Rate your hunger before:
1 2 3 4 5 6 7 8 9 10 (10 = famished)
Rate your hunger after:
1 2 3 4 5 6 7 8 9 10 (1 = totally satisfied)

DESSERT OR SNACK #3:
TIME EATEN:

_____

_____

DAILY WATER (check boxes; aim for sixteen 8-oz glasses):

☐ ☐ ☐ ☐ ☐ ☐ ☐ ☐ ☐ ☐ ☐ ☐ ☐ ☐ ☐ ☐

EXERCISE
DATE: _____

MORNING ENERGIZER:

Check option A ☐ , or option B ☐

Strength Training (list exercises):
repetitions / sets

_____

_____ / _____

_____

_____ / _____

_____

_____ / _____

_____

_____ / _____

_____

_____ / _____

**OPTIONAL CARDIO INTERVAL
OR OTHER PHYSICAL ACTIVITY:**

_____

_____ / _____

_____

_____ / _____

DAY 6

DATE: _____

BREAKFAST:

_____

_____

Rate your hunger before:
1 2 3 4 5 6 7 8 9 10 (10 = famished)

Rate your hunger after:
1 2 3 4 5 6 7 8 9 10 (1 = totally satisfied)

SNACK #1:

_____

_____

Rate your hunger before:
1 2 3 4 5 6 7 8 9 10 (10 = famished)

Rate your hunger after:
1 2 3 4 5 6 7 8 9 10 (1 = totally satisfied)

LUNCH:

_____

_____

Rate your hunger before:
1 2 3 4 5 6 7 8 9 10 (10 = famished)

Rate your hunger after:
1 2 3 4 5 6 7 8 9 10 (1 = totally satisfied)

SNACK #2:

_____

_____

Rate your hunger before:
1 2 3 4 5 6 7 8 9 10 (10 = famished)
Rate your hunger after:
1 2 3 4 5 6 7 8 9 10 (1 = totally satisfied)

DESSERT OR SNACK #3:
TIME EATEN:

_____

_____

DAILY WATER (check boxes; aim for sixteen 8-oz glasses):

☐ ☐ ☐ ☐ ☐ ☐ ☐ ☐ ☐ ☐ ☐ ☐ ☐ ☐ ☐ ☐

EXERCISE
DATE: _____

MORNING ENERGIZER:

Check option A ☐ , or option B ☐

Strength Training (list exercises):
repetitions / sets

_____

_____ / _____

_____

_____ / _____

_____

_____ / _____

_____

_____ / _____

_____

_____ / _____

OPTIONAL CARDIO INTERVAL
OR OTHER PHYSICAL ACTIVITY:

_____

_____ / _____

_____

_____ / _____

DAY 7

DATE:_____

BREAKFAST:

_____

_____

Rate your hunger before:
1 2 3 4 5 6 7 8 9 10 (10 = famished)
Rate your hunger after:
1 2 3 4 5 6 7 8 9 10 (1 = totally satisfied)

SNACK #1:

_____

_____

Rate your hunger before:
1 2 3 4 5 6 7 8 9 10 (10 = famished)
Rate your hunger after:
1 2 3 4 5 6 7 8 9 10 (1 = totally satisfied)

LUNCH:

_____

_____

Rate your hunger before:
1 2 3 4 5 6 7 8 9 10 (10 = famished)
Rate your hunger after:
1 2 3 4 5 6 7 8 9 10 (1 = totally satisfied)

SNACK #2:

_____

_____

Rate your hunger before:
1 2 3 4 5 6 7 8 9 10 (10 = famished)

Rate your hunger after:
1 2 3 4 5 6 7 8 9 10 (1 = totally satisfied)

DESSERT OR SNACK #3:
TIME EATEN:

_____

_____

DAILY WATER (check boxes; aim for sixteen 8-oz glasses):

☐ ☐ ☐ ☐ ☐ ☐ ☐ ☐ ☐ ☐ ☐ ☐ ☐ ☐ ☐ ☐

EXERCISE
DATE: _____

MORNING ENERGIZER:

Check option A ☐ , or option B ☐

Strength Training (list exercises):
repetitions / sets

_____

_____ / _____

_____

_____ / _____

_____

_____ / _____

_____

_____ / _____

_____

_____ / _____

OPTIONAL CARDIO INTERVAL
OR OTHER PHYSICAL ACTIVITY:

_____

_____ / _____

_____

_____ / _____